CARDIOVASCULAR PHYSIOLOGY

AN INTEGRATIVE APPROACH

CARDIOVASCULAR PHYSIOLOGY

AN INTEGRATIVE APPROACH

Evelyn M. Scott

MANCHESTER UNIVERSITY PRESS

Copyright © Evelyn M. Scott 1986

Published by
Manchester University Press, Oxford Road, Manchester M13 9PL, UK
27 South Main Street, Wolfeboro, New Hampshire 03894-2069, USA

British Library cataloguing in publication data

Scott, Evelyn M.
    Cardiovascular physiology: an integrated
    approach. —— (Studies in integrated
    physiology)
    1. Cardiovascular system
    I. Title II. Series
    612'.1   QP102

Library of Congress cataloging in publication data applied for

ISBN 0 7190 1776 9 hardback
      0 7190 1807 2 paper

Printed in Great Britain by
Robert Hartnoll (1985) Ltd
Bodmin Cornwall

CONTENTS

PREFACE

I decided to write this book as a result of my experiences in teaching undergraduates and, in particular, medical students who read physiology as part of their pre-clinical course.

It has three main aims. Firstly to teach students the principles involved in cardiovascular physiology. All too often students become submerged by the details of the subject and, in doing so, seemingly fail to grasp the underlying and important concepts. In an attempt to remedy this, I have emphasised the more important concepts and their relative importance to each other.

Secondly, I have included an up-to-date account of the control of the cardiovascular system which is intended to replace the outdated accounts of the vasomotor centre found in most textbooks. Since most of this material is taken from original papers or specialist reviews, it is by its nature not readily accessible to undergraduates or to non-specialists in the field. For this reason I have made the account of control rather more comprehensive than would normally be needed, by, for example, preclinical medical students.

Thirdly, I have discussed what happens to the cardiovascular system under different circumstances. This again is an important area which students often find difficult to understand.

The book also includes references to the possible clinical significance of the mechanisms I have described. There is also a chapter devoted to the techniques used to assess the functioning of the cardiovascular system and its control mechanisms in man.

The book is aimed mainly at undergraduates taking a course in physiology at universities and polytechnics and particularly those studying physiology as part of their medical degree. In addition, since it contains an up-to-date review of the subject, it should hopefully be useful for teachers of biological sciences at universities, polytechnics and sixth forms who are not necessarily specialists in cardiovascular physiology, but who wish to bring themselves up-to-date in the subject.

Acknowledgements

I am grateful to many colleagues for their most helpful comments on specific chapters of earlier drafts particularly, in Manchester, to Professors Case and Green and Drs. Rutishauser, Waterhouse and Watt and Mr. E. Kirkman in the Department of Physiology; to Professor H.B. Stoner and Dr. R.A. Little of the MRC Trauma Unit; to Dr. D. Rowlands of the Department of Cardiology at Manchester Royal Infirmary; in Leeds, to Professor B. Jewell and Dr. M. Boyett in the Department of Physiology and Dr. R. Hainsworth in the Department of Cardiovascular Studies, and in London to Professor L.H. Smaje at Charing Cross Hospital Medical School and Professor K.M. Spyer at the Royal Free Hospital Medical School.

However, of course, any omissions or errors in the text remain my responsibility.

I would also like to express my thanks to Mrs. M. Hagan for typing the manuscript and to Mrs. S. Millward for producing the diagrams.

HAEMODYNAMICS OF THE CIRCULATION

1.1 Introduction

Micro-organisms, in which the surface area to volume ratio is high, can obtain the oxygen and nutrients necessary for life from the surrounding fluid by simple diffusion through their external membrane. Waste products are removed by the same route. In larger animals, simple diffusion through the surface of the animal is inadequate to supply the necessary oxygen to the tissues and thus specialised systems have evolved which serve this function.

In mammals, the supply of oxygen to the tissues and the removal of carbon dioxide from the tissues are the functions of the respiratory and cardiovascular systems. The transfer of gases still takes place by simple diffusion but the site of this exchange — the lungs — is within the body. Since gases cannot diffuse from the atmosphere into the lungs at a sufficiently high rate, air is drawn in by the action of the respiratory muscles. It then enters a series of tubes, the bronchi and bronchioles, which end in blind sacs, called alveoli — the site of gas exchange. The exchange of oxygen and carbon dioxide between air and blood is by simple diffusion. This process is optimised by the huge surface area of the alveoli and the proximity of the blood vessels to the air in the alveoli. Blood is specialised for the transport around the body of a range of substances including oxygen, carbon dioxide, nutrients, hormones and anti-infection agents.

1.2 General arrangement of vessels in the circulation

Blood is pumped around the body through two separate circuits arranged in series. One circuit, the systemic circulation, distributes blood to the bulk of the body's tissues, and the other, the pulmonary circulation, pumps blood through the lungs so that exchange of gases can occur. These two circuits are very similar. Each consists of a pump and a network of distributing vessels, the arteries. Arteries give rise to vessels whose function is to regulate blood flow — the arterioles, vessels where exchange occurs — the capillaries, and a network of collecting vessels — the venules and veins. The properties of the pulmonary circulation do, however, differ in some ways from those of the systemic circulation, as will be discussed in Section 6.1.

The heart consists of four chambers, the right and left atria and the right and left ventricles. The ventricles are the main pumps, contraction of the atria contributing to the filling of the ventricles. (For further details of the structure of the heart, see Chapter 2, Figure 2.1). De-oxygenated blood from the systemic circulation enters the right atrium via the veins and then passes to the right ventricle. When the muscle in the wall of the right ventricle contracts, blood is forced into the pulmonary artery and hence passes to the

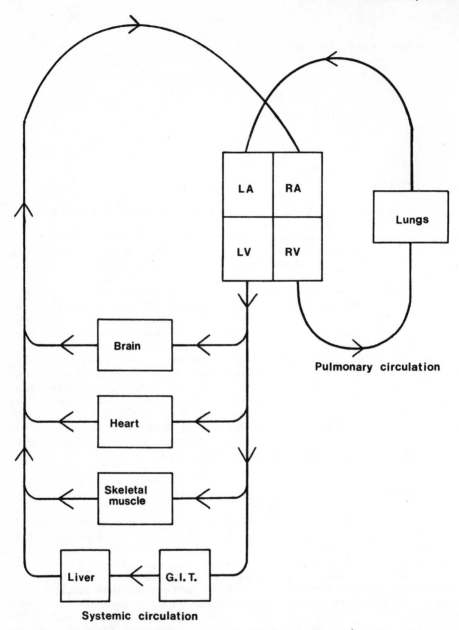

Figure 1.1. Diagrammatic representation of the heart and circulation to show the pulmonary circulation and the systemic circulations (e.g. to brain, heart and muscle). Also shown on the systemic side of the circulation is an example of a portal circulation where blood travels to the gastro-intestinal tract and to the liver before returning to the heart. LA, left atrium; LV, left ventricle; RA, right atrium; RV, right ventricle.

lungs where the transfer of gases occurs. Oxygenated blood then passes back via the pulmonary veins to the left atrium and then into the left ventricle. Contraction of the left ventricle forces blood into the aorta from whence it is distributed via the arteries around the body to the capillaries, which are the site at which exchange with the tissues occurs. De-oxygenated blood then returns to the right atrium. In the systemic circulation, arteries contain oxygenated blood and veins de-oxygenated blood, whereas in the pulmonary circulation, the reverse is true.

Thus, the pulmonary and systemic circulations are arranged in series. Within the systemic circulation, the vessels supplying the different organs and tissues are arranged in a parallel fashion. This arrangement has the advantage that flows to different regions can be varied independently to suit the requirements of that tissue at any particular time.

In general, the arrangement of blood vessels is such that blood travels along the arteries and arterioles to the capillaries where exchange occurs and then back to the heart via the veins. However, in some circulations there are two sets of capillaries in series, and the existence of this second set of capillaries is related to the different functions that organs have to perform. The presence of this second set of capillaries is termed a portal system. Portal systems are found in the gastro-intestinal tract, the kidney and supplying the pituitary gland in the brain.

Within the gastro-intestinal tract, blood flows from the stomach and intestines to the liver via a portal system before returning to the heart. This allows the liver to remove toxic materials before they enter the general systemic circulation and to remove foodstuffs for storage.

The portal system supplying the anterior part of the pituitary gland allows the trophic hormones to be secreted by the hypothalamus into the vessels connecting the hypothalamus and pituitary gland. Thus, these trophic hormones can act specifically at one site, rather than being released into the general circulation where their concentration would be very small. This portal system also reduces the time taken for the hormones to have their effects, reduces their breakdown in the blood and eliminates any widespread effects that would result from their release into the systemic circulation.

Within the kidney, the presence of a portal system allows fluid to be filtered from the blood at a high pressure and then at a later stage, when the pressure within the vessels is lower, allows the filtrate to be modified by reabsorption and secretion. The second capillary network allows a large net uptake of substances by reabsorption.

1.3 Energetics of the circulation

Fluids, including blood, will flow from one site to another if the total fluid energy at the one site exceeds that at the other. There are three components of fluid energy:

(1) Pressure energy;
(2) Gravitational potential energy;
(3) Kinetic energy.

Changes in gravitational potential energy do not directly affect the force which drives the blood from one point to another but they do have important effects on the circulation. This can best be understood by considering hydrostatic pressure. In the horizontal posture, the hydrostatic pressures in the arteries of the different parts of the body are approximately equal. Similarly, the hydrostatic pressures in the veins in the different parts of the body are approximately equal. However, when a subject stands up, there is an increase in the hydrostatic pressures in all the vessels below the heart and a decrease in the hydrostatic pressures in vessels above the level of the heart. These changes in hydrostatic pressures in the different vessels will depend upon their distance from the heart. For example, when a man 1.8 m in height stands, his feet will be about 1.2 m below the level of his heart. Therefore, the hydrostatic pressure in the vessels of his feet will increase by an amount given by pgh, where p is the density of blood, g is the acceleration due to gravity and h is height. In SI units $p \approx 10^3$ kg·m^{-3}, $g = 9.8$ m.s^{-2}, $h = 1.2$ m; hence pressure $= 10^3$ x 9.8 x 1.2 Pa $= 11.76$ kPa ≈ 88 mmHg.

Since the total fluid energy remains the same, these changes in posture do not directly affect the blood's driving force, but they do, in some vessels, change the pressure across the vessel walls (the transmural pressure). In the vessels of the feet, this increase in transmural pressure will lead to distension of the vessels. This distension will be particularly marked in the veins, since they are thinner-walled and more distensible than the arteries (see Section 4.2.4). When vessels are situated within strong fascial sheaths or in fluid-containing cavities, such as the abdomen or brain, transmural pressures are less affected by postural changes, since pressures both inside and outside the vessel will alter and thus the pressure across the wall (the transmural pressure) will be less affected.

The contribution to the total fluid energy made by the kinetic energy varies within different parts of the circulation and also between rest and exercise. In the atria and pulmonary artery, kinetic energy makes a significant contribution to total fluid energy (about 12 per cent) at rest and is very important when cardiac output is increased, as it is during exercise. For example, when cardiac output is increased three-fold, kinetic energy makes up 50 per cent of the total fluid energy in the atria and pulmonary artery. In the systemic arterial system, the kinetic energy factor is negligible at rest and is only significant in the aorta during heavy exercise.

1.3.1 *Determinants of laminar blood flow*

At rest, blood flow from the root of the aorta through to the right atrium is determined by the difference in pressure between these two vessels (P_1 - P_2) and the resistance to blood flow (R):

$$\text{Blood flow} = \frac{(P_1 - P_2)}{R}$$

1.3.1.1 *The Hagen—Poiseuille equation.* The factors affecting the resistance to flow of a Newtonian fluid such as water in a rigid tube are described in the Hagen—Poiseuille equation:

$$\text{Flow} = \pi r^4 \frac{(P_1 - P_2)}{8 l \eta}$$

where r and l are the radius and length of the vessel respectively and η is the viscosity of the liquid.

Thus, increases in the pressure difference along the vessel (the perfusion pressure or driving pressure) or in the radius of the vessel will result in an increase in flow, whereas increases in the length of the vessel or the viscosity of the liquid will decrease flow. The relationship between the flow and the fourth power of the radius of the vessel is important because it shows that halving the radius of the blood vessel will result in a sixteen-fold increase in the resistance to blood flow. The mechanisms by which the radius can be altered are discussed in detail in Chapter 5.

1.3.1.2 *Influence of viscosity.* According to the Hagen–Poiseuille equation, the resistance to flow is also affected by the viscosity of the fluid. However, blood is not a Newtonian fluid, since it is made up of a suspension of cells in plasma. The viscosity of blood depends upon the haematocrit (the percentage of the blood volume taken up by the cells), the velocity of blood flow, the diameter of the blood vessels and the temperature. Thus, the viscosity of blood varies within the circulation, so we refer to the regional viscosity when discussing the flow of blood through particular vessels within the circulation. When the haematocrit is low, for example in anaemia, viscosity is low so resistance will fall and flow will increase; in conditions such as polycythaemia, where the haematocrit is increased, viscosity is high so resistance will increase.

At low velocities of blood flow, cells appear to be arranged in an irregular fashion within the blood. However, as the velocity of flow increases, the cells become orientated in a regular manner towards the centre of the stream, leaving a layer of plasma in contact with the vessel wall. This reduces the frictional forces between the plasma and cell portions so the viscosity at higher flow rates is lower than that at lower flow rates. This dependence of viscosity on blood flow means that when the initial rate of blood flow is low an increase in blood flow will result in a fall in viscosity and therefore a fall in the resistance to blood flow.

Providing that the flow rate is reasonably high, the viscosity of blood drops progressively when the diameter of the blood vessels decreases below 200–300 μm; this is known as the Fåhraeus–Lindqvist effect. This effect is not seen with plasma and so must be due to the presence of cells within the blood. Thus, the radius of a vessel has an important effect on the viscosity of the blood flowing through it. In small-diameter capillaries, the viscosity of blood is almost the same as that of plasma. Many explanations have been offered to explain this effect. One is that when blood vessels branch, 'plasma skimming' may occur; that is, smaller branches will contain a greater proportion of plasma than is found in the larger vessels. Plasma skimming may be a consequence of the positioning of blood cells towards the centre of the vessels, assuming that the thickness of the plasma layer remains constant. The secretion of a substance from the endothelium of the capillaries which lowers viscosity has also been suggested as a cause. The Fåhraeus–Lindqvist effect means that changes in the radius of small blood vessels do not change flow as much as would be predicted from the Hagen–Poiseuille equation. For example, if a vessel dilates, blood flow does not increase by the amount predicted by the fourth power of the change in radius because blood viscosity rises causing a diminution in blood flow. At slow flow rates, the changes in viscosity which result from changes in the rate of blood flow predominate over the Fåhraeus–Lindqvist effect.

The Fåhraeus–Lindqvist effect probably largely explains the fact that the viscosity of the blood when measured *in vivo* is lower than the values obtained *in vitro*. Other factors which will cause regional differences in viscosity when blood flow is low are the aggregation of red cells and the plugging of capillaries by white blood cells. Temperature will also influence the viscosity of the blood: when the fingers are cooled in iced water, regional viscosity may increase three-fold or more.

1.3.2 *Turbulent flow*

The Hagen—Poiseuille equation assumes that flow is streamline or laminar. Under certain circumstances, blood flow may become turbulent, that is, the cells are no longer orientated in a regular fashion towards the centre of the stream but rapid, radial mixing of the different components occurs. The occurrence of turbulence can be predicted by estimating the Reynolds number (Re). The Reynolds number is determined by the equation

$$Re = \frac{vd\rho}{\eta}$$

where v is the average velocity of blood flow, d is the diameter of the tube, ρ is the density and η the viscosity. Turbulence is likely to occur when the Reynolds number exceeds 2000. Thus, turbulence is more likely to occur when blood has a high velocity of flow, a low viscosity and when the vessel is of large diameter. In addition to these factors, turbulence will also develop when there are abrupt variations in the dimensions of the vessels or irregularities in the vessel walls.

Turbulence develops gradually; when blood flow is turbulent, the increased friction between molecules leads to a greater kinetic energy loss. Blood flow then becomes proportional to the square root of the pressure drop along the vessel, rather than directly proportional to the pressure drop as it is when blood flow is laminar. Thus, to produce turbulent flow, a pump such as the heart has to do considerably more work than it would have to do in order to produce the same laminar flow.

Turbulent flow occurs within the chambers of the heart and this is important in mixing the venous blood from different parts of the body. Turbulent flow may also occur within the aorta. In a healthy subject, blood flow in the smaller vessels is laminar. This is because as the vessels branch, their total cross-sectional area increases and therefore the average velocity of flow decreases. Furthermore, the diameters of the vessels will also fall. Both these factors will result in a reduction of the calculated Reynolds number.

In pathological states, such as when plaques are formed within vessels, turbulent flow may occur within the peripheral circulation. In this case, the plaques induce turbulence at and just beyond the site where the vessel is occluded. When a vessel is obstructed, turbulence occurs at a very much lower value of the Reynolds number than is normal in a long straight vessel.

Turbulence is usually accompanied by vibrations which can be heard. The appearance of turbulent flow in the circulation is the basis of the normal method of measurement of blood pressure in man (see Section 10.1.2). In this technique, the turbulent flow is produced by mechanically occluding the blood vessel. Structural changes which result in a narrowing of vessels, or of the orifices of the heart, may also result in the appearance of turbulent flow which can be detected as a 'murmur'. In conditions such as severe anaemia, where the viscosity of the blood is reduced, and there is a compensatory increase in the rates of blood flow, murmurs can also be heard.

Turbulent flow, as well as increasing the work of the heart, also increases the likelihood of the development of blood clots or thrombi. This may occur when heart valves are replaced by artificial valves. It is therefore important when designing such valves that care be taken to avoid the development of turbulent flow and so of thrombi.

Further reading

Burton, A.C. (1968). *Physiology and Biophysics of the circulation.* Year Book Medical Publishers, Chicago.

2

THE ELECTRICAL AND MECHANICAL PROPERTIES OF THE HEART

When considering the physiology of the heart and its relationship to structure, it is important to bear in mind the considerable task that the heart has to perform as a pump. Firstly, it must pump continually and in the correct sequence approximately 70 times every minute for perhaps 70 years. Yet, at the same time, the rate and force of its contractions must be capable of very fine regulation so that the output of the heart can be adjusted to fit the needs of the body. The structure and arrangement of the components of the heart are well suited to the functions they have to perform.

2.1 Structure of the heart

The heart is made up of two thin-walled atria and two thicker-walled ventricles, the latter separated by the interventricular septum. (See Figure 2.1.) The wall of the left ventricle is thicker than that of the right ventricle, which has to do less work since it is pumping against a lower pressure. The atria and ventricles are joined by the fibrous atrio-ventricular septum or AV ring, which is penetrated by the tricuspid valve on the right and the mitral or bicuspid valve on the left. These valves between atria and ventricles consist of three triangular flaps (or cusps) on the right side and two on the left side of the heart. These cusps are thick at the valve ring but at their free borders they are thinner and quite flexible, and it is here that they are attached to papillary muscles via the chordae tendinae. These papillary muscles originate from inside the ventricles, and are often used in the study of cardiac muscle because their muscle fibres are arranged in a more parallel fashion than is normally found in the heart. There are also valves between the left ventricle and the aorta and between the right ventricle and the pulmonary artery called semi-lunar valves. Each consists of three cusps or flaps of tissue.

2.1.1 *Ultrastructure of cardiac muscle*
Normal cardiac muscle fibres are cylindrical and branched, approximately 100–150 μm long and 15–25 μm in diameter. They are surrounded by a membrane, the sarcolemma, which is made up of the plasma membrane of the cell and connective tissue. Intercalated discs are present between the muscle fibres. These consist of the two opposing cell membranes and the intercellular space. The structure of these intercalated discs varies but the intracellular or sarcoplasmic surface of the membrane is often reinforced by a thick layer of filaments. The branching of the muscle fibres and the low resistance to current flow offered by the intercalated discs means that when one cell is excited action potentials spread generally and quickly. Thus, large parts of the heart can function as a syncytium, even though structurally there is no continuity between the muscle fibres. Because of the presence of the fibrous atrio-ventricular septum the atria and the ventricles act as two functional· syncytia.

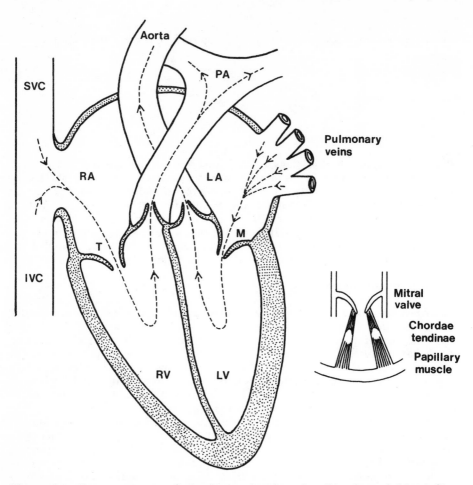

Figure 2.1. Gross anatomy of the heart showing the direction of blood flow through the heart. Insert is a magnified diagram of the mitral valve to show the attachments of the chordae tendinae. SVC, superior vena cava; IVC, inferior vena cava; RA, right atrium; RV, right ventricle; PA, pulmonary artery; LA, left atrium; LV, left ventricle; M, mitral valve; T, tricuspid valve.

Within each fibre are myofilaments which contain contractile proteins as well as normal cellular components. These myofilaments are not organised into clearly circumscribed myofibrils as they are in skeletal muscle. Instead they form a single large bundle which fills most of the muscle fibre. The myofilaments consist of a series of repeating structures (approximately 2 μm in length), the sarcomeres. The sarcomere is the contractile unit of the heart and changes in its length cause muscle contraction. The arrangement of molecules within the sarcomeres has been found from studies using the electron microscope. Sarcomeres are delineated from each other by dark lines, the Z lines, and between the Z lines are alternate dark and light bands (see Figure 2.2). The central A band contains both thick and thin filaments and the lighter I band on either side of the A band contains only thin filaments.

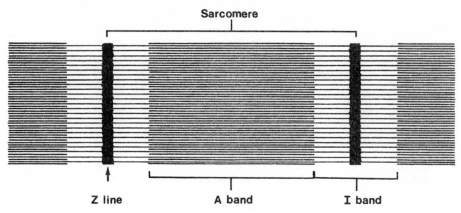

Figure 2.2. The arrangement of filaments within a papillary muscle.

The thick filaments contain only the protein myosin whereas the thin filaments contain the protein actin and various regulatory proteins such as troponin and tropomyosin. The structural arrangement of the components within the myofilaments allows the rapid development of tension within the cardiac muscle (see Section 2.5).

Lying close to the myofilaments is a system of transverse tubules (T-tubules) and the sarcoplasmic reticulum (see Figure 2.3). The transverse tubules in

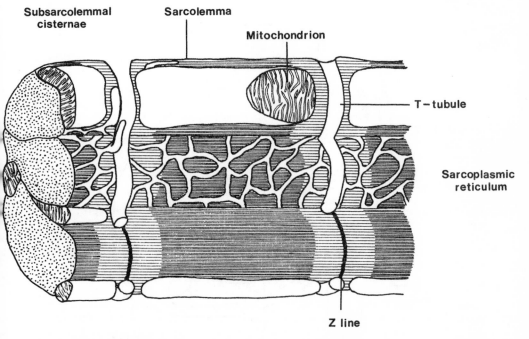

Figure 2.3. The arrangement of T-tubules and sarcoplasmic reticulum within mammalian cardiac muscle (From Fawcett & McNutt, 1969.)

cardiac muscle are larger than those found in skeletal muscle. They are continuous with the cell surface and extend to the sarcomeres at the Z line. There are also numerous longitudinal connections between the T-tubules. The sarcoplasmic reticulum of cardiac muscle is less extensive than that of skeletal muscle. It is composed of a simple plexus of tubules of rather uniform calibre which freely anastomose along the myofilaments. In cardiac muscle, there are no terminal cisternae arising from the sarcoplasmic reticulum as are found in skeletal muscle. However, there are small sacular expansions of the reticulum called subsarcolemmal cisternae (see Figure 2.3) which are in close contact with either the T-tubules or the sarcolemma at the periphery of the fibre.

2.2 Initiation and conduction of electrical activity in the heart

Even when the nerves to the heart are cut, the heart will continue to beat in a rhythmic manner. This is because the heart contains specially modified cells which are responsible for the initiation of the heart's spontaneous electrical activity and its conduction through the different chambers of the heart, as well as cells concerned with muscular contraction.

This electrical activity is normally initiated in an area of the heart called the sinu-atrial node or SA node (see Figure 2.4) which is situated near the junction of the superior vena cava and the right atrium. The cells within the SA node are modified cardiac muscle cells which are thinner than normal and receive a rich innervation from the vagal and sympathetic nerves.

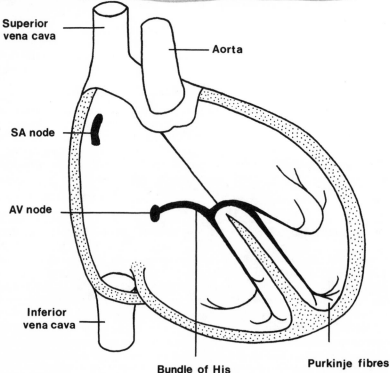

Figure 2.4. The arrangement of the specialised conducting tissues in the heart.

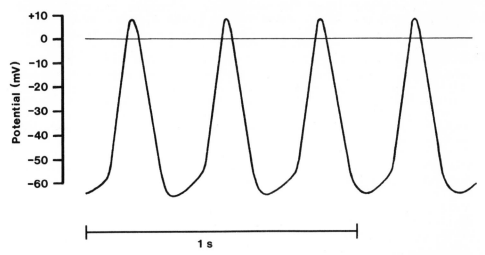

Figure 2.5. Spontaneous potential changes recorded from the SA node of a rabbit to show pacemaker activity (From Noble, 1969.)

2.2.1 *The pacemaker potential*
When recordings are made of the membrane potentials of cells in the SA node, they show at rest a spontaneous depolarisation — the pacemaker or pre-potential (see Figure 2.5). When the depolarisation is sufficient to bring the membrane potential to threshold level an action potential is produced. The resting membrane potential of the cells in the SA node is about -60mV. The initial depolarisation during the pacemaker potential results from a slow decline in the permeability of the membrane to potassium. This is followed by a later inward depolarising current which, in the cells of the SA node, is thought to be carried mainly by calcium ions. Both the fall in potassium permeability and the rise in the permeability to calcium result in a depolarisation of the membrane. Beyond threshold, depolarisation is due to a rapid increase in the permeability of the cell to sodium and, in the SA node cells, a further influx of calcium ions may be important. Repolarisation is a result of a fall in permeability to both calcium ions and sodium ions and an increase in the permeability of the membrane to potassium ions.

2.2.2 *The conduction of electrical activity*
The action potentials initiated at the SA node spread out through the atrial muscle but their speed of conduction is greater when they travel through particular bundles of the atrial fibres. There is some disagreement as to whether these muscle bundles contain specialised cells similar to those found in the SA node. The atrio-ventricular or AV node and the Bundle of His to which it gives rise are the only muscle connections between the atria and the ventricles. They both contain cells which are specialised for conduction. The fibres in the AV node are smaller than normal muscle fibres (approximately 7 μm in diameter). Their action potentials are small and slow and there are few nexi between the cells so electrical activity does not pass readily from cell to cell. For these reasons, cells in the AV node conduct more slowly (0.03 — 0.05 m·s^{-1}) than normal cardiac muscle fibres. This results in a delay at the AV node, which is important because it allows atrial contraction to be completed

before the ventricles start to contract.

The electrical activity then passes down a bundle of specialised fibres, the Bundle of His, to the ventricular muscle. The fibres within the Bundle of His, the Purkinje fibres, are arranged in strands approximately 50 μm in diameter. The electrical activity is conducted very rapidly (4 m·s^{-2}) along the fibres, which run below the endocardial surface of the ventricular muscle to the different parts of the ventricles. From the Bundle of His the electrical activity is transmitted to the interventricular septum and then through the ventricular muscle from the endocardial surface to the epicardial surface. The speed of conduction through the ventricular muscle is very much less than that through the Bundle of His. The rapid spread of electrical activity to the different parts of the ventricles allows them to contract almost synchronously.

Unsteady membrane potentials, or pacemaker potentials, are found only in the cells which are specialised for the initiation and conduction of electrical activity through the heart, that is, cells within the SA node, the AV node and the Purkinje fibres. The ionic mechanisms responsible for pacemaker activity in Purkinje fibres differ from those in SA node cells. The resting membrane potential of Purkinje cells is greater (-90 mV) than that found in SA node

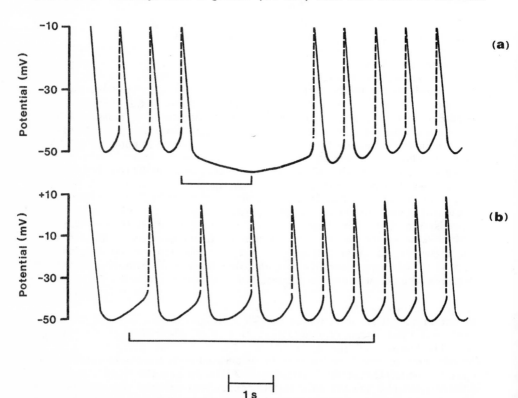

Figure 2.6. Pacemaker activity recorded during stimulation of the autonomic nerves to the heart.
(a) The effect of stimulation of the vagal nerve (indicated by the horizontal line) and
(b) The effect of stimulation of the sympathetic nerves (indicated by the horizontal line) (From Hutter & Trautwein, 1956.)

cells. In Purkinje cells the pre-potential is thought to result at least partly from an increase in the permeability of the cell to sodium ions, rather than to calcium ions as is the case in the SA node. In both types of cell, the fall in potassium permeability contributes to the pacemaker activity.

2.3 Control of cardiac rhythm and conduction

The intrinsic rate of firing of the cells in the SA node can be altered by a number of factors. The dense autonomic innervation of the SA node is important in regulating the slope of the pre-potential. Vagal stimulation reduces this slope and also hyperpolarises the membrane (see Figure 2.6a). These changes are thought to be the result of a rise in the permeability of the membrane to potassium, thus increasing the rate at which potassium ions leave the cell. Stimulation of the sympathetic nerves to the SA node results in an increase in the slope of the pre-potential (see Figure 2.6b), thus reducing the time taken for the cell to reach threshold. This change is thought to be due to a decrease in the permeability of the membrane to potassium ions and an increase in the permeability of the cell to calcium ions. Stimulation of the sympathetic nerves also speeds up conduction of electrical activity through the conducting system. Conversely, vagal stimulation causes a marked reduction in the conduction velocity through the AV node.

Heart rate increases during inspiration and decreases during expiration. As will be discussed in Section 8.2.2, this change in heart rate with respiration, which is termed sinus arrhythmia, results from changes in the rate of discharge of the vagal and sympathetic nerves innervating the SA node.

Increases in temperature and stretching the SA node both increase the rate of spontaneous depolarisation of the membrane. There is a change in heart rate of approximately 10 beats·min^{-1} for each 1°C increase in temperature. Stretching the SA node results in an increase in heart rate up to a critical point when further stretching results in a slowing of the heart.

Normally the sequence of electrical events occurring in the heart is governed by the SA node. This is because cells of the SA node reach threshold more quickly so have a faster intrinsic rhythm than cells in other parts of the conducting system. Thus electrical activity arrives at the other parts of the conducting system before their cells have depolarised to threshold. In the event of destruction of the SA node alone, the fastest-firing group of cells will take over. Normally, these are the cells in the AV node so the intrinsic rhythm of the heart will be slower. In the event of destruction of the AV node alone, electrical activity cannot pass through from the atria to the ventricles. Under these circumstances, the Purkinje fibres will initiate the electrical activity in the ventricles, the atrium continuing to be governed by the faster rate of firing of the SA node.

2.3.1 *Arrhythmias*

Irregularities in the rate, rhythm or sequence of depolarisation of cardiac cells are termed arrhythmias. Some arrhythmias occur because of the activity of ectopic foci. (Any piece of cardiac tissue, when damaged or ischaemic, may become a pacemaker, either temporarily or permanently; such sites are termed ectopic foci). The cells in ectopic foci initiate waves of electrical activity which spread across the heart and give rise to additional contractions which are termed extrasystoles. If, as in the atrium, the rate of discharge from these ectopic foci is very rapid, then a tachycardia of as much as 250–300 beats·min^{-1} may occur. If the contractions are co-ordinated, this is termed flutter.

The existence of flutter can also be explained by the re-entry theory. Waves of excitation can spread away from pacemaker tissue along circular pathways. If the length of these pathways is short, then the impulse will arrive back at the starting point while the cells are refractory and therefore the activity will die out. In diseased hearts, however, this electrical activity may arrive back at the starting point after the refractory period is over so the impulse will be repropagated. This can occur: (*a*) if the length of the pathway is increased, as will occur if the heart is dilated; (*b*) if the rate of conduction is slowed; or (*c*) if the refractory period of the cells is shortened. Both (*b*) and (*c*) can be brought about by drugs or may occur in the diseased heart.

If these movements of electrical activity are along regular pathways, then flutter will occur. However, the electrical activity may travel in an irregular fashion across the whole of the atrium or ventricle, leading to very high-frequency unco-ordinated contractions. This is called fibrillation. Ventricular fibrillation can also occur if there are large differences in the speed at which electrical activity is conducted through the Purkinje system. Again, if the conduction velocity is reduced or the refractory period of the Purkinje cells is reduced, then electrical activity may be repeatedly repropagated leading to extra unco-ordinated contractions. Normally, such abnormal repropagation is prevented by the fast speed of conduction in the conducting system and the long duration of the Purkinje fibre action potentials.

As will be discussed later in this chapter, atrial contraction is not essential for life, but if fibrillation occurs in the ventricular muscle, blood can no longer be ejected from the ventricle, and death will result.

2.4 The cardiac muscle action potential

Normal cardiac muscle fibres, that is fibres without specialised conducting or pacemaker properties, have steady resting potentials, as have skeletal muscle cells. The spread of depolarisation through the heart results in a depolarisation of these cardiac muscle cells and, ultimately, in contraction.

The action potentials of cardiac muscle are of longer duration than those of skeletal muscle or nerve. The duration of the cardiac action potential may be as much as 500 ms compared to, perhaps, 2 ms in skeletal muscle. In the heart, the duration of the action potential varies very much between cells from different areas of the heart, ventricular action potentials being longer than atrial action potentials. This long duration is because of the presence of a plateau phase (see Figure 2.7*a*), where depolarisation is prolonged.

The existence of different 'gating mechanisms' in the membrane, whose level of activation may vary both with time and with the voltage across the membrane, can be used to explain the complex nature of the cardiac action potential (Figure 2.7*b*). In non-pacemaker tissues, the initial fast depolarisation of the membrane beyond threshold is due to a voltage-dependent increase in the permeability of the membrane to sodium ions, bringing the membrane towards the equilibrium potential for sodium. At the same time, depolarisation produces a sharp fall in the permeability of the membrane to potassium ions. The initial increase in sodium permeability is quickly stopped and the sodium permeability is restored towards, but not to, resting values. Because potassium permeability is low, this residual sodium current, which is insignificant in nerve action potentials, contributes significantly to the inward depolarising current and so helps to produce the plateau. The initial fast increase in sodium permeability is followed by a

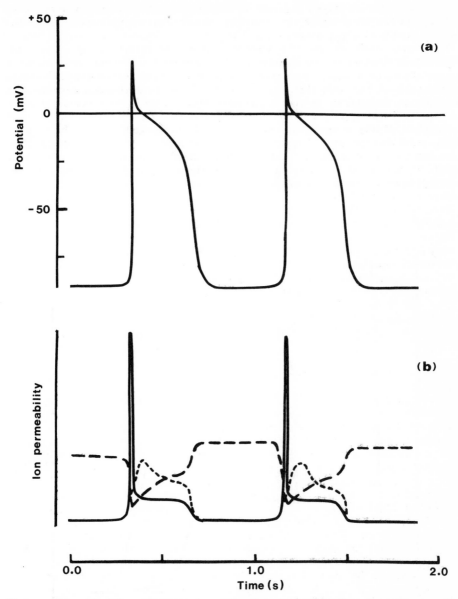

Figure 2.7. (a) The changes in potential and (b) the changes in the permeability of the membrane to sodium (——), calcium (---) and potassium (— —) ions which occur during an action potential in ventricular muscle.

slower increase in the permeability to calcium ions. Thus, the membrane is maintained in a state of depolarisation, the plateau, and this results in the duration of the action potential in cardiac muscle cells being much greater than that in skeletal muscle cells. Repolarisation is brought about by inactivation of this slow increase in the permeability to sodium and calcium combined with a delayed increase in the permeability of the membrane to potassium. These permeability changes return the membrane towards the equilibrium potential for potassium.

The long duration of the cardiac action potential is of functional importance because it prevents the cardiac muscle from being tetanised — a lethal state for a pump. Figure 2.8 shows the action potential of a cardiac muscle cell on the same time scale as a recording of the tension developed in a papillary muscle. In cardiac muscle the absolute refractory period, that is, the period during which no action potential can be generated by the cell regardless of the strength of the stimulus, is prolonged. As can be seen in Figure 2.8, the absolute refractory period has still not been completed after the tension has reached its peak and has started to decline. Thus, a further contraction cannot be superimposed upon the peak tension of the previous contraction and tetanus cannot occur.

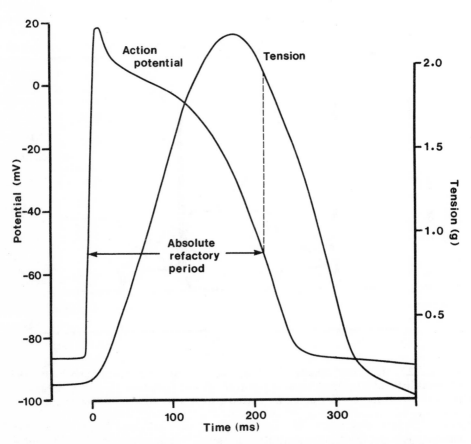

Figure 2.8. The changes in potential and the changes in tension which occur during a single cardiac contraction recorded from a papillary muscle.

2.5 The mechanism of muscle contraction

In cardiac muscle, contraction is thought to occur by the formation of linkages or cross-bridges between actin and myosin molecules and the subsequent sliding of the thin (actin) and thick (myosin) filaments over each other. This sliding filament hypothesis, also explains how contraction takes place in skeletal muscle. The chemical energy required to form the cross-bridge attachments is provided by the hydrolysis of the terminal phosphate on the ATP molecule by the ATPase present in the myosin head.

Between contractions, the formation of cross-bridges between the actin and myosin molecules is prevented by the presence of the regulatory proteins troponin and tropomyosin. Troponin is bound to tropomyosin, and is distributed at intervals along the actin strands. The troponin—tropomyosin complex blocks the formation of cross-bridges between myosin and actin. This inhibition is removed by calcium ions, thus allowing contraction to occur.

2.6 Excitation—contraction coupling

Following the initiation of electrical activity in the heart, depolarisation of the sarcolemma of the muscle fibre is rapidly conducted along the T-tubules, and this causes the release of intracellular calcium, mainly from the sarcoplasmic reticulum (see Figure 2.3). It is generally accepted that the release of calcium from the sarcoplasmic reticulum is triggered by the entry of calcium into the cell during the plateau phase of the action potential (see Section 2.4). Some workers also maintain that calcium is released purely in response to the depolarisation of the sarcolemma.

In mammalian hearts, the first 150—200 ms of the action potential is important in releasing intracellular calcium. Calcium attaches to the troponin molecule. Tropomyosin then moves to expose the site on the actin which attaches to the myosin and thus crossbridge formation can occur. Simultaneously, the calcium causes the activation of the ATPase on the myosin head. This ATPase provides the energy for contraction by breaking down ATP.

The process of excitation—contraction coupling can be modified at a number of stages causing the force of contraction of cardiac muscle to vary.

The amount of calcium released from the sarcoplasmic reticulum will depend upon the duration of the action potential. Changes in the duration of the cardiac action potential are most commonly associated with changes in the frequency of contraction; the duration normally becoming less as the frequency increases.

The stores of calcium within the sarcoplasmic reticulum have to be replenished with calcium from outside the cell. A number of different channels and pumps is involved in transporting calcium across the cell membrane. One mechanism which is particularly important is the sodium—calcium exchange mechanism linking the transport of sodium ions out of the cell and the transport of calcium ions into the cell. Because of the existence of this exchange mechanism, an increase in extracellular sodium levels hinders the entry of calcium into the cell and an increase in intracellular sodium enhances the uptake of calcium by the cell. Factors which influence the activity of the sodium—potassium pump will alter the intracellular and extracellular concentration of sodium ions and consequently of calcium ions. For example, cardiac glycosides, which slow the rate of activity of the sodium—potassium pump, will result in an increase in the intracellular concentration of sodium. This will increase the uptake of calcium by the sarcoplasmic reticulum and thus increase the amount of calcium available for release.

There is also evidence that the sensitivity of the contractile proteins to calcium varies. Changes in sensitivity occur with changes in sarcomere length and also with variations in the amount of phosphorylation at several sites on the protein. This phosphorylation also modifies the rate of re-uptake of calcium by the sarcoplasmic reticulum and the amount of force produced by a given degree of activation. It is not yet known whether these changes occur on a beat-to-beat basis but it is known that the phosphorylating reactions are sensitive to cyclic AMP and calcium and that the sarcoplasmic concentration of these substances will alter on a beat-to-beat basis.

2.7. Events of the cardiac cycle

The sequence of electrical events in the heart is important in that it determines the sequence of mechanical events occurring within the different chambers of the heart. Changes in electrical activity in the heart cause the development of potential differences, which, when suitably amplified, can be recorded from electrodes on the surface of the body. A fuller account of the electrocardiogram or ECG is given in Section 10.2.1 but a brief mention is required here so that the electrical events can be correlated with the mechanical events. The waves of the ECG are: the P wave, representing atrial depolarisation, the QRS complex representing ventricular depolarisation and within which the effects of repolarisation of the atria are hidden, and the T wave which represents repolarisation of the ventricles (Figure 2.9*d*).

The mechanical events can best be described by referring to the changes in pressure which occur in the different chambers of the heart during a single cardiac cycle (see Figure 2.9*a*). Changes in the pressure in the different chambers of the heart can be accurately measured by inserting cannulae into the heart which are attached to pressure manometers (see Section 10.2.3).

In a normal subject, blood will flow through the heart from atria to ventricles to arteries. Flow occurs along a pressure gradient and can be affected by the opening and closure of the valves between the atria and ventricles and the ventricles and the aorta or pulmonary artery. These valves normally allow flow in one direction only. The AV valves will open when the pressure in the atria exceeds that in the ventricles and will close when pressure in the ventricles exceeds that in the atria. Retrograde flow is prevented by the chordae tendinae. Similarly, the semilunar valves will open when pressure in the ventricles exceeds that in the aorta or pulmonary artery and will close when pressure in the aorta or pulmonary artery exceeds that in the ventricles.

In the following discussion the events occurring on the left side of the heart will be described. Those occurring on the right side of the heart are similar but the pressures developed are lower (see Section 6.1).

At the start of the cardiac cycle, both the atrium and ventricle are relaxed and blood is flowing from the veins into the atrium and then into the ventricle through the open AV valve. Filling of the ventricle is largely passive and occurs in two phases, an initial rapid period of filling lasting for about 0.1 s following opening of the AV valves, and a period of slower filling during the middle part of diastole.

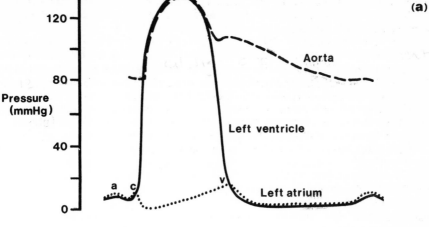

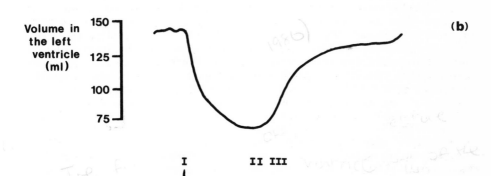

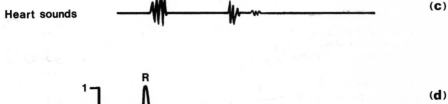

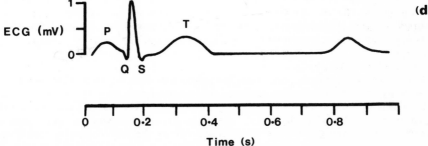

Figure 2.9. (a) The changes in pressure in the aorta (---), left ventricle (——) and left atrium (......); (b) the changes in volume in the left ventricle, (c) the heart sounds and (d) the electrocardiogram (ECG) during a single cardiac cycle.

The mechanical events are initiated by the spontaneous depolarisation of the SA node and the spread of electrical activity through the heart. As a result of this depolarisation of the atrium (represented by the P wave on the ECG) the atrium contracts. At rest, the duration of this contraction is about 0.1 s and its contribution to the filling of the ventricle is small; at rest only about 15 per cent of the ventricular filling takes place during atrial systole. Atrial systole may be of more functional significance in situations where venous return is increased, for example, during exercise, or when the passive filling of the ventricles is impaired. Atrial contraction and the relaxation which follows result in a rise and fall in the pressure within the atrium — often referred to as the 'a' wave on the atrial pressure pulse.

Meanwhile, the electrical activity has passed through the AV node and down the Bundle of His and depolarisation of the ventricles starts (as shown by the QRS complex on the ECG). Therefore, the ventricle starts to contract and, as it contracts, pressure in the ventricle rises and soon exceeds the pressure in the atrium, thus closing the mitral valve. The ventricle continues to contract. Because both the mitral and aortic valves are closed, this period of contraction is termed the period of isometric contraction. During this period, pressure within the ventricle rises steeply. As the ventricles start to contract, the closed AV valves bulge into the atrium causing a sharp rise in the atrial pressure. When pressure in the ventricle exceeds the pressure in the aorta, blood is ejected into the aorta. During ejection, the AV valves are pulled down and consequently pressure in the atrium falls sharply. The rise and fall in atrial pressure forms the 'c' wave of the atrial pressure pulse.

The onset of ejection at first expands the aortic wall. There follows a period of rapid ejection and pressure within the aorta rises sharply. The rate at which blood is ejected then falls off. The rate at which aortic pressure declines is determined by the elasticity of the walls of the aorta and the rate at which the blood is removed from the aorta into the peripheral vessels. The total period of ventricular systole is about 0.3 s.

Repolarisation of the ventricular muscle then follows, as is shown by the T wave on the ECG. Ventricular pressure falls sharply as the ventricle relaxes, but the aortic pressure drop is less because of the elastic recoil of the walls of the aorta. The aortic valve shuts when the pressure in the ventricle is less than that in the aorta. The ventricular pressure continues to fall and this stage, because both the mitral and aortic valves are closed, is termed the period of isometric relaxation.

Throughout the cycle, blood has been returning to the heart via the veins and hence atrial pressure has been steadily rising, causing the rising phase of the 'v' wave of the atrial pressure pulse. When atrial pressure rises above ventricular pressure, the AV valves open, causing the falling phase of the 'v' wave, and the cycle recommences.

2.7.1. *Heart sounds*

Opening of the valves does not normally produce a detectable sound but closure of the heart valves is responsible for the heart sounds (see Figure 2.9c) which can be heard either by placing an ear on the chest wall or by using a stethoscope. Classically, there are four areas of auscultation where sounds and murmurs originating from the four heart valves are heard clearly (see Figure 2.10).

The first sound is commonly described as 'lubb'. It has a frequency of between 30 and 80 Hz and a duration of 0.05 s and it occurs during closure of the AV valves. It is produced partly by vibration of the AV valves and the

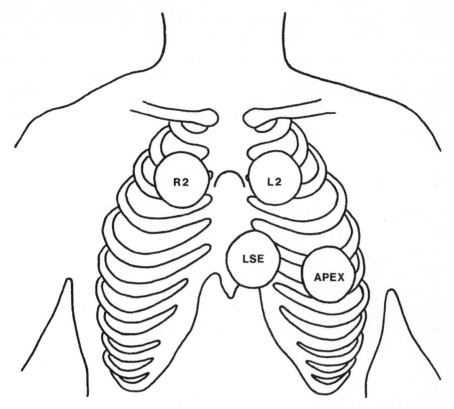

Figure 2.10. The four classical areas of auscultation on the chest wall; the second right intercostal space (R2), the second left intercostal space (L2), the lower left sternal edge (LSE) and the point of maximal impulse (APEX).

adjacent cardiac wall on closure of the valves and partly as a result of turbulent blood flow (see Section 1.3.2).

The second heart sound has a higher frequency (150–200 Hz) and a shorter duration (0.025s) and is commonly described as 'dup'. It is caused by closure of the aortic and pulmonary valves. The second heart sound is split into two sounds during inspiration. This is because as intrathoracic pressure falls during inspiration, venous return to the right side of the heart increases (see Section 4.3). This increase in filling will increase right ventricular stroke volume, thus increasing the length of right ventricular systole and delaying closure of the pulmonary valve. This coincides with a reduction in left ventricular stroke volume because of a decreased return of blood from the lungs which will result in the earlier closure of the aortic valve. The effects of respiration are more marked on the right side of the heart than on the left, and thus the changes in timing of pulmonary valve closure are greater than the changes in timing of aortic valve closure.

Two additional sounds, the third and fourth sounds, may be heard in some individuals. The third sound may be heard in healthy children and young adults during rapid ventricular filling and is caused by vibration of the cardiac walls. The fourth sound occurs during atrial systole but is not normally audible in health.

Additional sounds or murmurs may be heard. These are caused by excessive turbulence of blood in the heart. The murmurs may be present in normal healthy individuals without any cardiac disease and result from an increase in the velocity of blood flow through the heart. However, they may also result from a narrowing of the valves' apertures (stenosis) or the presence of faulty valves (incompetence) allowing the regurgitation of blood. Murmurs of differing characteristics and timings heard over different parts of the chest wall are a useful diagnostic aid in assessing cardiac disease, but are outside the scope of this book. The interested reader may find an account in any standard text of clinical cardiology.

Further reading

Fawcett, D.W. & McNutt, N.S. (1969). The ultrastructure of the cat myocardium. *Journal of Cell Biology*, **42**, 1–67.

Noble, D. (1979). *The Initiation of the Heartbeat*. 2nd ed. Clarendon Press; Oxford.

Parmley, W.W. & Talbot, L. (1979). The heart as a pump. In: *Handbook of Physiology, Section 2, The Cardiovascular System*, Volume 1, *The Heart* (ed. R.M. Berne), pp. 429–60. American Physiological Society; Bethesda.

Winegard, S. (1979). Electromechanical coupling in heart muscle. In: *Handbook of Physiology, Section 2, The Cardiovascular System*, Volume 1, *The Heart*, pp. 393–428. American Physiological Society; Bethesda.

3

MECHANISMS CONTROLLING THE OUTPUT OF THE HEART

In this chapter I shall discuss the mechanisms whereby the amount of blood pumped out of the heart every minute can be varied, and consider how these different mechanisms operate in the intact heart. Changes in the output of the heart can be achieved either by changing the rate at which the heart beats or by changing the force of contraction of the cardiac muscle.

Changes in the rate at which the heart contracts are achieved by changing the slope of the pacemaker potential of the cells in the SA node (see Section 2.3).

3.1 Control of the force of contraction of cardiac muscle

Changes in the force with which cardiac muscle contracts can be brought about by two mechanisms:

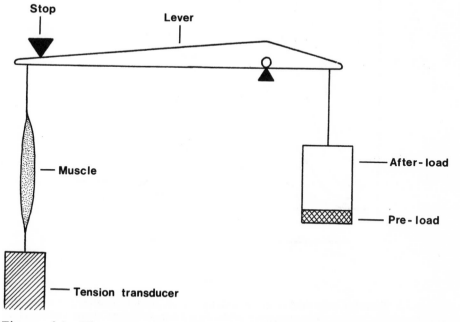

Figure 3.1. The apparatus used to investigate isometric and isotonic contractions of cardiac muscle. The muscle is bathed in oxygenated Ringer's solution and stimulated electrically. (From Sonnenblick, 1962).

(1) by altering the initial length of the muscle fibres;
(2) by mechanisms other than those which change the initial length of the
      muscle fibres — inotropic effects.

These two mechanisms can most easily be demonstrated by looking at the
properties of isolated cardiac muscle. Much of this work has been done using
the papillary muscle from the heart. This preparation has the advantage of
being relatively thin and, thus, less likely than a thicker piece of tissue to
become hypoxic. In addition, the fibres within the muscle tend to be arranged
in a more parallel fashion than those in the main body of the heart.

Various models have been constructed to aid our understanding of the way
in which cardiac muscle contracts. In most of these models the cardiac muscle
is seen as having a contractile element and elastic components.

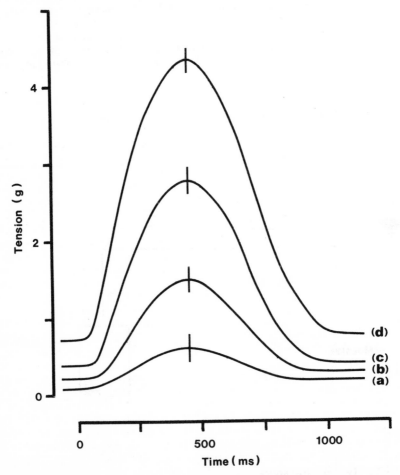

Figure 3.2. Records obtained from a cat papillary muscle showing four single
isometric muscle twitches superimposed. The four twitches were obtained at
initial lengths of (a) 8.5, (b) 9.0, (c) 9.5 and (d) 10 mm. The vertical bars
represent the peak tension reached during each twitch. (From Sonnenblick,
1962.)

Cardiac muscle, like skeletal muscle, can contract both isometrically and isotonically. During an isometric contraction, for example, when the ventricle is contracting but both the mitral and aortic valves are closed, the length of the muscle remains constant but the tension will increase. During an isotonic contraction, for example, when blood is ejected from the ventricle, the muscle will shorten. Both isometric and isotonic contractions can be demonstrated in the papillary muscle preparation. The muscle is attached at one end to the end of a lever and at the other end to a tension transducer (see Figure 3.1). The length of the muscle can be altered by making it support different loads before it starts to contract. The application of these loads prior to contraction (referred to as pre-loads) will stretch the muscle. It is also possible to arrange that the muscle meets a load in the course of a contraction — this load is called the after-load. During an isometric contraction the lever is fixed and thus shortening cannot occur (see Figure 3.1). During an isotonic contraction the lever is free and thus the muscle is able to shorten. In both types of contraction the contractile element will shorten. During an isometric contraction the elastic elements will become stretched, tension will rise and the overall length of the muscle will not alter. In an isotonic contraction, initially as the contractile element contracts the elastic elements will become stretched. In this initial stage, the muscle develops tension but its overall length stays relatively constant. When the tension developed is sufficient to enable the load to be lifted, then further contraction of the contractile element will result in shortening of the muscle.

3.1.1 *Effect of changes in the initial length of muscle fibres*
Using this preparation it is possible to show the effects of changes in the pre-load, which will change the initial length of the muscle fibres, on an isometric contraction. Figure 3.2 shows the effect of increasing the length of the muscle by 0.5 mm increments. The changes in the tension developed at rest (the resting or passive tension) and the tension developed during a contraction (the active tension) as a result of increasing the length of the muscle are both shown graphically in Figure 3.3. It can be seen that the initial stretching of the muscle results in an increase in both the resting tension and the active tension. However, a stage is reached where further increases in the length of the muscle, although causing resting tension to continue to rise, cause no further increase in active tension. Similar relations between resting and active tension and the length of the muscle are found in skeletal muscle.

Changing the initial length of cardiac muscle results in changes in the force of contraction of the muscle by two different mechanisms. Firstly, the length of the muscle will determine the degree of overlap between the thick and thin filaments. As discussed in Section 2.5, it is the formation of cross-bridges between myosin and actin molecules and the subsequent sliding of the thick and thin filaments against each other which results in contraction of the muscle. At short muscle lengths these actin and myosin filaments are not aligned along their whole length. The actin filaments may overlap each other or may be compressed at their ends. As the muscle is stretched, an optimum length is reached at which the degree of overlap between the actin and myosin filaments is maximal and at this point, the active tension developed by the muscle during contraction will be maximal (see Figure 3.3). Further stretching will result in a reduction in the overlap between the filaments and thus a reduction in the active tension developed by the muscle.

Changes in the lengths of the muscle fibres have also been shown to influence the sensitivity of the contractile element to calcium (see Section 2.6) and thus the force with which the muscle contracts.

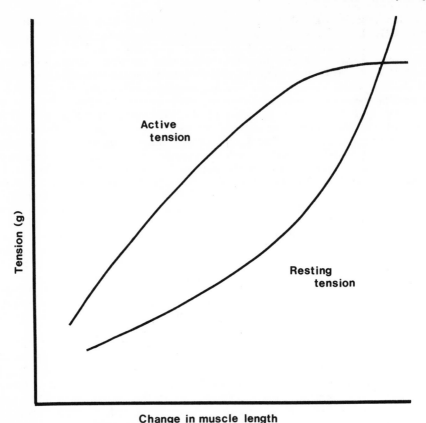

Change in muscle length

Figure 3.3. The changes in resting tension and active tension which result from increasing the length of a strip of cardiac muscle.

The observation that the force of contraction of cardiac muscle depends on the initial length of the muscle fibres is very important and is the basis of Starling's law of the heart (see Section 3.2.3).

3.1.2 *Effect of inotropic agents*

Using the same papillary muscle preparation, inotropic effects (changes in the force of contraction from the same initial muscle length) can also be demonstrated, as shown in Figure 3.4. In this record two isometric contractions are shown. Twitch (*a*) is a contraction recorded under control conditions and twitch (*b*) is a contraction recorded at the same muscle length as (*a*), but when noradrenaline has been added to the solution bathing the muscle. Noradrenaline does not affect the resting tension but does increase the tension developed during the contraction (the active tension). Noradrenaline also increases the rate at which the muscle contracts and relaxes and thus decreases the duration of the contraction. In the intact heart, this reduction in the duration of systole produced by noradrenaline is important, as will be discussed later in this chapter.

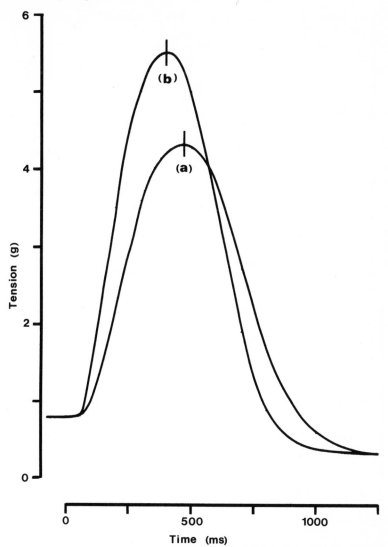

Figure 3.4. Records obtained from a cat papillary muscle showing two single muscle twitches, recorded at the same initial length, superimposed. The vertical bars represent the peak tension reached during each twitch.
Twitch (*a*) was recorded under control conditions and
Twitch (*b*) was recorded when noradrenaline has been added to the solution bathing the muscle such that the concentration was 0.5 μg·ml^{-1} of bathing fluid. (From Sonnenblick, 1962.)

Catecholamines, such as noradrenaline and adrenaline, modulate the force of contraction of cardiac muscle by affecting excitation–contraction coupling. These effects are mediated by the excitation of β-adrenergic receptors in the heart. Catecholamines increase the inward current carried by calcium ions during the cardiac action potential (see Section 2.4) and this would be expected to increase the amount of calcium released by the sarcoplasmic reticulum.

β-adrenergic receptor activation also results in the phosphorylation of the troponin molecule, decreasing its sensitivity to calcium ions. However, the net effect of β-adrenergic receptor activation is to produce a pronounced increase in the force of contraction of cardiac muscle.

3.1.3 *Effect of changes in the after-load*
The effect of changes in the after-load on the contraction of cardiac muscle can also be determined by using a papillary muscle preparation. In this case the lever (see Figure 3.1) is free and the muscle is able to shorten and lift the load. Thus, using this preparation, the velocity of shortening of the muscle at different loads can be obtained (see Figure 3.5). It can clearly be seen that as the load increases the velocity of shortening of the muscle decreases, i.e. the muscle can move light loads more quickly than heavier loads.

3.1.4 *Effects of changes in the frequency of contraction*
The force of contraction of cardiac muscle is also determined by the frequency of contraction. Assuming that there is an adequate supply of oxygen, increases in the frequency of stimulation will result in an increase in the force of contraction — the so-called treppe or Bowditch staircase effect.

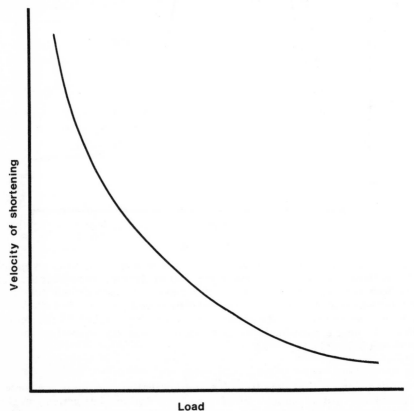

Figure 3.5. The relationship between the velocity of shortening of cardiac muscle and the load on the muscle.

In the heart, a longer-than-normal delay between beats or a pause after an additional beat (or extrasystole) will also be followed by a stronger contraction. These effects of changing the frequency of contraction are probably mediated by altering the number of calcium ions available to the muscle cells.

Thus, in an isolated cardiac muscle preparation, the force of contraction is determined by the initial length of the muscle (the pre-load), the load that the muscle has to contract against (the after-load), the presence of inotropic agents, its temperature and the interval between contractions. It is these same factors which will determine the force of contraction of the intact heart, as will be discussed in the rest of this chapter.

3.2 Control of cardiac output

The volume of blood pumped out by the heart every minute is called the cardiac output. Details of how the cardiac output can be measured in man are given in Section 10.2.4. Values of about 5 litres every minute are normally quoted for the cardiac output in conscious man at rest, but like all physiological 'normal' values, there is a range of normal values which varies with the size, age, sex and posture of the individual and with the time of day.

Long-term, cardiac output must be equal to venous return. Over a time-course of a few beats, the left heart is able to 'milk' from the reservoir of blood in the pulmonary circulation (see Section 6.1) but over a longer period of time, output (that is, cardiac output) and input (that is, venous return) must be matched. Thus, in the following account of the regulation of the output of the heart, the factors influencing the return of blood to the heart (see Section 4.3) must also be considered.

Cardiac output is defined as the product of the heart rate (the number of times the heart beats every minute) and the stroke volume (the volume of blood ejected with each beat of the heart). At rest, the heart rate is normally about 70 beats·min^{-1} and the stroke volume about 70 ml per beat.

3.2.1 *Control of heart rate*

As has been discussed earlier (see Section 2.2), the heart is capable of beating spontaneously. Normally, however, it is also influenced by external factors (see Section 2.3). The SA node receives an innervation from both sympathetic nerves — the ansae subclaviae, and parasympathetic nerves — the vagal nerves. The sympathetic nerves, particularly the right ansa subclavia, act to increase the heart rate. Conversely, the parasympathetic nerves, particularly the right vagal nerve, act to slow the heart rate. At rest, in the young adult, both the sympathetic and parasympathetic nerves to the heart are tonically discharging but the actions of the parasympathetic nerves predominate. When all the nerves to the heart are cut, the heart rate increases to 100–120 beats·min^{-1}.

There are other factors which will alter heart rate: an increase in the level of circulating adrenaline or noradrenaline results in an increase in heart rate, as do increases in temperature, some drugs and stretching the SA node (see Section 2.3).

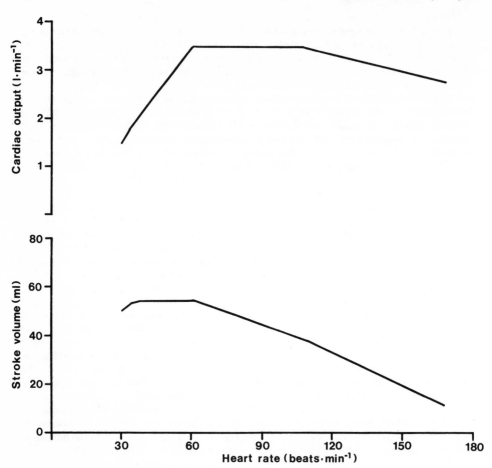

Figure 3.6. The effects of changes in heart rate on the stroke volume (bottom) and the cardiac output (top) in the dog. (From Miller *et al.*, 1962.)

3.2.2 *Effects of changes in heart rate*
It might seem from the equation

$$\text{cardiac output} = \text{heart rate} \times \text{stroke volume}$$

that an increase in either the heart rate or the stroke volume will result in an increase in the cardiac output. In fact, these two variables do not change independently; changes in the heart rate may affect the stroke volume. Studies have been carried out in animals to show the effect of changes in heart rate on both the stroke volume and the cardiac output. In these experiments the AV node was blocked so that the normal passage of impulses from the atria to the ventricles was prevented, and the ventricular muscle was stimulated directly at different frequencies (see Figure 3.6). Increases in heart rate from the very low intrinsic rate of the ventricles to about 60 beats·min⁻¹ did not affect the stroke volume. Therefore, since heart rate increased but stroke volume remained constant, cardiac output increased markedly. Further increases in heart rate up to about 100 beats·min^{-1} resulted in decreases in stroke volume. Thus, since heart rate increased but stroke volume decreased, cardiac output either remained constant or fell slightly. Further increases in heart rate over 150 beats·min^{-1} resulted in much larger falls in stroke volume and falls in cardiac output. Measurements in conscious animals of the volume of blood contained in the ventricles at the end of filling (end-diastolic volume) have provided evidence for a reduction in filling when the heart rate is increased.

Thus, except in situations in which the heart rate initially is very low, increases in heart rate, without an associated positive inotropic effect, will result in a fall in stroke volume. If this fall in stroke volume is sufficiently great, it will result in a fall in the cardiac output. The reason for this is that when heart rate increases, the period of a single cardiac cycle will be reduced. Since the time taken for the muscle to contract (systole) will remain much the same, the time for filling (diastole) will shorten considerably. At high heart rates, this reduction in the duration of diastole will become even more significant because there will be an encroachment upon the period of rapid filling of the ventricle. Thus, if the time available for filling of the heart is inadequate, the stroke volume will fall. When filling is compromised, as it will be when the heart rate is very high, then the contribution to filling of the ventricle made by atrial contraction will become more significant than it is under resting conditions.

Increases in heart rate alone without an associated increase in the force of contraction of the cardiac muscle do occur under both physiological and pathological circumstances. For example, stimulation of atrial receptors (see Section 7.2.1) will result in an increase in heart rate with no associated positive inotropic effect.

Thus, when heart rate increases, instead of assuming that this will result in an increase in the cardiac output, we ought to be looking for mechanisms which are responsible for maintaining the stroke volume in the face of a reduction in the diastolic filling time. These mechanisms have been discussed in section 3.1 and can be divided into (*a*) changing muscle length and (*b*) inotropic effects on the heart muscle. In the following section the way in which these mechanisms operate in the intact animals will be discussed.

3.2.3 *Control of stroke volume*
Starling's law of the heart states that the energy of contraction of cardiac muscle is dependent on the initial length of the muscle fibres, and can be demonstrated in man when the heart is *in situ*. Here, we can record the pressure in the left ventricle at the end of filling or diastole (left ventricular end-diastolic pressure, LVEDP) and use this as an index of the initial length of the muscle fibres. It has been shown that when the length of the muscle fibres is measured, changes in their length are related to LVEDP and that this relationship remains unaltered during stimulation of the sympathetic nerves. Instead of relating stroke volume to LVEDP, stroke work (the product of the stroke volume and the aortic pressure) is normally used. This is because changes in the aortic pressure, the after-load on the muscle, will also affect the force of contraction (see Section 3.1.3).

Figure 3.7 shows the way in which stroke work varies with LVEDP. Stroke work increases linearly with increases in LVEDP over a range of values for LVEDP up to about 15 cmH$_2$O. Beyond this, further stretching of the muscle (that is, further increases in LVEDP) does not result in an increase in the stroke work. The shape of this curve shown in Figure 3.7 resembles the length—tension curve obtained in isolated cardiac muscle as shown in

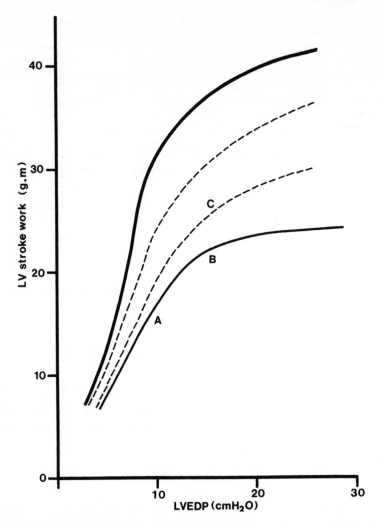

Figure 3.7. The relationship between left ventricular stroke work and left ventricular end-diastolic pressure (LVEDP). The lower unbroken line represents control data, the upper unbroken line represents results obtained during maximal stimulation of the left stellate ganglion and the two dotted lines represent results obtained during two levels of submaximal stimulation. (modified from Sarnoff *et al.*, 1960.) See text for a discussion of A, B and C.

Figure 3.3. *In vivo*, these increases in the length of the muscle fibres will result from an increase in venous return. Thus as venous return increases, the right ventricle will contract more strongly and its output will increase.

This mechanism is also important in maintaining equal the outputs from the two sides of the heart. If there is an increase in the filling of either ventricle, then that ventricle will contract more strongly and its output, too, will be increased. Thus, stroke volume may be increased by increasing the filling of the heart — the end-diastolic volume.

The second way in which stroke volume may be increased is to increase the force of contraction of the cardiac muscle so the heart empties more completely; stroke volume is increased because the volume remaining in the left ventricle at the end of systole (left ventricular end-systolic volume, LVESV) is reduced. If the sympathetic nerves are stimulated, the relationship between left ventricular stroke work and LVEDP can again be described (see Figure 3.7). It can be seen that, again, as LVEDP increases, up to a point, stroke work will also increase. In addition, at any given LVEDP, indicating a given muscle length, sympathetic stimulation results in an increase in the stroke work. The upper unbroken line in Figure 3.7 shows the effect of maximal sympathetic stimulation. At lower frequencies of stimulation, curves will be recorded lying between the two as shown by the dotted lines in Figure 3.7. Thus, it is often said that there is a family of Starling curves.

It can now be seen that changes in stroke volume can be produced either by changes in the initial length of the muscle, that is, by moving along one of the Starling curves (e.g. from A to B on Figure 3.7), or by inotropic agents, that is, by moving from one curve to another (e.g. from B to C on Figure 3.7). In heart failure, it is thought that the reduced force of contraction results from a movement from a higher curve to a lower curve rather than just from an overstretching of the muscle fibres in the heart.

Increasing the force of contraction of cardiac muscle by a positive inotropic effect, such as by stimulation of the sympathetic nerves, has two important advantages compared with increasing the force of contraction by increasing the initial length of the muscle. Firstly, since inotropic agents increase the velocity of contraction and of relaxation, the duration of systole is reduced and thus the time available for filling is increased. Secondly, since stimulation of the sympathetic nerves results in a more complete emptying of the heart, rather than an increase in the filling of the heart, the heart will be comparatively smaller. According to the law of Laplace (see Section 4.1), a reduction in the radius of the heart will result in a reduction in the tension developed in the walls at any given pressure and hence a reduction in the oxygen consumption of the heart (see Section 3.3).

The maximum rate of change of pressure within the left ventricle (dP/dt max) has been shown to be a sensitive index of inotropic effects on the heart. This index has the advantage of being simple and relatively easy to measure. Changes in the LVEDP, that is, changes in the initial length of the muscle, do not significantly alter this index. However, stimulation of the sympathetic nerves, particularly the left ansa subclavia, or infusion of catecholamines, both produce significant increases in dP/dt max (see Figure 3.8). These are by far the most important inotropic agents under physiological conditions. Stimulation of the vagal nerves results in a negative inotropic effect on the atrium but no physiologically significant negative inotropic effect on the ventricular muscle. Some workers have suggested that the vagal nerves may exert a negative inotropic effect on the ventricular muscle but, when controlled measurements of dP/dt max are made in normal animals, little or no effect is seen. It may be that, in more pathological situations, the vagal nerves do exert an influence on the ventricular muscle.

Increases in heart rate and aortic pressure also produce small positive inotropic effects on the heart. In the intact heart the small increase in the force of contraction due to increased frequency is far outweighed by the deleterious effect on the stroke volume of increasing the heart rate, and hence reducing the filling time (see Section 3.2.2). Similarly, increases in aortic pressure (the after-load) produce small positive inotropic effects on the heart (the Anrep effect). As can be seen from Figure 3.8, the inotropic effects

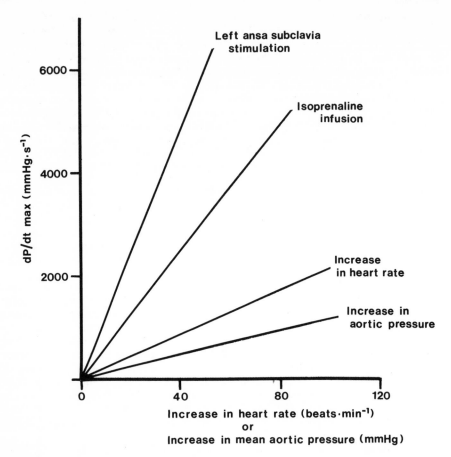

Figure 3.8. Effects of stimulation of the left ansa subclavia, infusion of isoprenaline (a catecholamine) and increases in heart rate and mean aortic pressure on the maximum rate of rise of pressure in the left ventricle (dP/dt max). (From Linden, 1968.)

of changes in heart rate and aortic pressure are very small compared with the effect of catecholamines on the heart.

Thus, in summary, the force of contraction of the heart can be varied in two ways. Firstly, when venous return increases, thus stretching the ventricular muscle fibres, the force of contraction of the heart will increase (Starling's law of the heart). Secondly, a number of interventions (of which the most important are changes in the activity in the sympathetic nerves and changes in the level of circulating catecholamines) will alter the force of contraction without changing the resting length of the muscle fibres (inotropic effects).

3.3 Cardiac work

The amount of oxygen used by the heart will vary depending on its activity. At rest the oxygen consumption of a normal heart is between 8 and 10 $ml \cdot min^{-1} \cdot 100$ g of $tissue^{-1}$. When the heart is stopped, but the coronary blood flow is maintained artificially, the oxygen consumption falls to about 2 $ml \cdot min^{-1} \cdot 100$ g^{-1}.

Since the major work of the heart is to pump a fluid against a pressure head, the external work done by the ventricle per beat is considered to be the

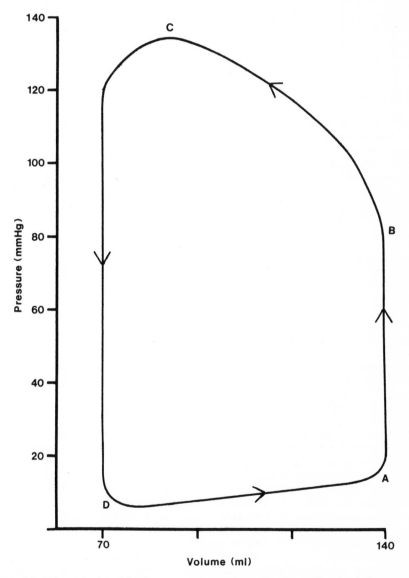

Figure 3.9. The relationship between pressure and volume in the left ventricle during a single cardiac cycle. See text for a discussion of A—D.

product of the stroke volume and the mean aortic pressure against which the heart is pumping. This disregards the kinetic factor, which will be considered later in this section. The external work done by the left ventricle can be expressed graphically by means of the pressure—volume diagram (see Figure 3.9). Point A represents the point at which filling of the ventricle is completed. At rest, the volume within the ventricle at this point is approximately 140 ml. Between A and B the ventricles are contracting isometrically and the pressure rises sharply. At B the pressure in the ventricle exceeds that in the aorta and blood is ejected into the aorta from the ventricle, hence the volume within the ventricle will fall between B and C. Between C and D the ventricle is relaxing and thus the pressure is falling. When the pressure in the ventricle falls below that in the aorta the aortic valve closes and therefore the volume within the ventricle will remain unchanged from this point until point D when the mitral valve opens. Between D and A the ventricle is filling with blood from the atrium and thus both pressure and volume will increase. Details of these events are given in Section 2.7.

The area within the curve ABCD has been used to estimate the external work done by the ventricle during each beat. Thus, either a doubling of the pressure or of the volume would be expected to produce an equal change in the external work done by the ventricle.

However, external work is also done in ejecting the blood from the ventricles into the aorta (kinetic energy). This kinetic energy is defined by the term $\frac{1}{2}mv^2$ where m is the mass of blood ejected from the ventricle and v is the velocity with which it is ejected. At rest only about 2—4 per cent of the useful work performed by the heart is in the form of kinetic energy. However, at high cardiac outputs, for example during exercise, the kinetic component can account for up to half the total external work done by the heart.

If the oxygen consumption of the heart was related only to the mechanical work the heart performed, then, increases in heart rate, stroke volume or aortic pressure would be expected to alter oxygen consumption in a predictable way. However, measurements of the amount of oxygen actually used by the heart under different circumstances show that the oxygen consumption of the heart is not simply related to the work done by the heart as calculated from the pressure—volume loop. If the external work done by the heart is increased by a rise in aortic pressure, this produces a much greater increase in the heart's oxygen consumption than is produced by a similar increase in external work due to an increase in stroke volume. Increases in heart rate also result in a very pronounced increase in the oxygen consumption of the heart in excess of that predicted from the increase in external work. These results occur because most of the oxygen consumed by the heart is used in developing tension within the heart rather than in the performance of external work.

For our understanding of how the heart functions the important observations are: firstly, that both increases in aortic pressure and heart rate result in a greater increase in the oxygen need of the heart than does an increase in stroke volume; secondly, increases in stroke volume produced by inotropic agents require a smaller increase in oxygen consumption than do equal increases in stroke volume resulting from increasing the length of the muscle fibres. This is because inotropic effects reduce the size of the heart and thus according to the law of Laplace (T α PR, see Section 4.1) the wall tension and consequently the oxygen consumption of the heart will be reduced. These observations have particular significance in situations when the supply of oxygen to the heart may be restricted as it is in patients with coronary artery disease (see Section 6.2).

Further reading

Brady, A.J. (1979). Mechanical properties of cardiac fibres. In: *Handbook of Physiology*, Section 2, *The Cardiovascular System*, Volume 1, *The Heart*, pp. 461–74. American Physiological Society: Bethesda.

Linden, R.J. & Snow, H.M. (1974). The inotropic state of the heart. In: *Recent Advances in Physiology*, 9th Edn. ed. R.J. Linden, Churchill Livingstone: Edinburgh.

STRUCTURE AND FUNCTION OF BLOOD VESSELS

In Chapter 1, I described the arrangement of the blood vessels in the circulation and considered the factors which influenced the flow of blood in tubes. In this chapter, I shall consider the structure and properties of the different vessels in the circulation.

4.1 Structural components of blood vessels

The walls of all the blood vessels, except the capillaries, are made up of three layers: an inner tunica intima, a middle tunica media and an outer tunica adventitia. The tunica intima is composed of a single layer of endothelial cells; the walls of capillaries consist of only this layer. The tunica media consists of smooth muscle and elastic tissue and the tunica adventitia is made up mainly of collagen and fibroblasts.

The role of the endothelial cells is to provide a smooth inner lining to the blood vessels and to offer a barrier which is selectively permeable to substances passing to and from the tissues.

The function of the elastic tissue is to produce an elastic tension in the walls of the vessels without expending biochemical energy. This elastic tension will resist the distending force which is applied to the walls of the blood vessels when the transmural pressure is increased. Blood vessels resist stretch more strongly the more they are stretched. By Laplace's law, the tension in the vessel wall (T) which opposes the stretch is directly related to the transmural pressure (P) and the radius of the vessel (R):

$$T \; \alpha \; PR$$

Thus, at a given radius, the pressure tending to distend the vessel is proportional and opposite to the tension in the wall which opposes the distension. If the distending pressure is increased the elastic tissue will be stretched and thus the wall tension will be increased and this will oppose further distension.

The collagen fibres in the tunica adventitia, also resist stretch. These fibres resist stretch much more than elastic fibres but, because of their rather loose arrangement within the vessel wall, they do allow vessels to distend to some extent.

The function of the vascular smooth muscle is to produce active tension in the wall of the vessel, thus reducing its calibre. The presence of elastic tissue in vessel walls allows contraction of the smooth muscle to produce graded changes in the calibre of the vessels. For example, in a vessel which contained no elastic tissue, an increase in transmural pressures would not cause a concomitant increase in the wall tension and thus the radius of the vessel would increase. At the new, larger radius, an even larger wall tension would be needed to oppose the increase in transmural pressure and thus the vessel would continue to distend until eventually the wall ruptured. This dilatation of the vessel wall is termed an aneurysm. Further, if vessels contained no elastic tissue, contraction of the smooth muscle in the wall would lead to an increase in the wall tension which would overcome the transmural pressure and lead to a reduction in the radius of the vessel and, hence, to closure of the vessel. Thus, the presence of elastic tissue allows the gradation of the diameter of the vessels as a result of changes in the force of contraction of the smooth muscle in the walls.

Vessels which have smooth muscle but very little elastic tissue in their walls, for example, the arteriovenous (A-V) anastomoses or shunts in the skin (see Section 6.5) tend to be either fully open or closed. The calibre of these vessels is extremely sensitive to changes in the active tension exerted by the smooth muscle in the walls. Other vessels which have a small amount of elastic tissue in their walls have a tendency to close when the distending pressure is low and the active tension is high. Closure occurs when either the pressure falls below a critical value or the wall tension increases above a critical value. This phenomenon, termed 'critical closure of blood vessels', may occur, for example, following a haemorrhage (see Section 9.1), where there is a fall in transmural pressure and an associated increase in active tension developed in the wall due to the reflex activation of the sympathetic vasoconstrictor fibres innervating the vessels.

4.2 Structure and properties of the different vessels

The pressures recorded within the different vessels of the circulation (see Figure 4.1) are related to their structure and function.

When the heart is not contracting, during the period of diastole, pressure within the left ventricle is approximately equal to atmospheric pressure. During contraction of the heart muscle, the period of systole, pressure within the ventricles rises to approximately 120 mmHg.

4.2.1 *Aorta and large arteries*
From the left ventricle, blood first enters the aorta and its large branches. The walls of these vessels contain a large amount of elastic tissue within the tunica media. During systole, the blood ejected into the aorta distends the vessel wall. Potential energy is stored within the elastic tissues of the aorta during systole and during diastole this is converted to kinetic energy. This ability of the aortic walls to distend and then recoil results in a damping of the pulsatile pressure, so that pressure within the aorta varies only between about 80 and 120 mmHg. Hence the term sometimes applied to these vessels - windkessel vessels - a windkessel being an elastic pressure chamber frequently incorporated in a mechanical pumping system to smooth out the individual strokes of the pump. With ageing and other degenerative changes the aorta loses its elasticity and, thus, the change in pressure in the aorta with each cardiac cycle (the pulse pressure) increases in amplitude.

Passing down the arterial tree, the arteries become smaller and their walls contain less elastic tissue and more smooth muscle. These are termed the muscular arteries. The pulse pressure recorded in these vessels is much greater in amplitude than that recorded in the aorta.

4.2.2 *Arterioles and precapillary sphincters*

The greatest drop in pressure in the system occurs across the next group of vessels, the arterioles and precapillary sphincters. These vessels are the major site of resistance in the circulation.

The arterioles are the larger of the two groups (50–100 μm in diameter) and their tunica media contains two to four layers of smooth muscle. Their walls contain only a fragmented sheath of connective tissue between the endothelium and the tunica media instead of the layer of elastic tissue found in larger arteries (the internal elastic lamina). Changes in the diameter of the arterioles result in the diversion of blood from one region to another in the body. How this distribution of blood occurs and the mechanisms responsible for altering the calibre of these vessels are discussed in detail in Chapter 5.

In amphibians precapillary sphincters can be identified anatomically. These vessels are smaller than arterioles (10–15 μm) and have no elastic tissue remaining in their walls between the endothelium and the smooth muscle of the tunica media. However, in mammals, in most circulations, there are no anatomical sphincters present at the precapillary sites, although precapillary sphincters do exist in the hepatic circulation.

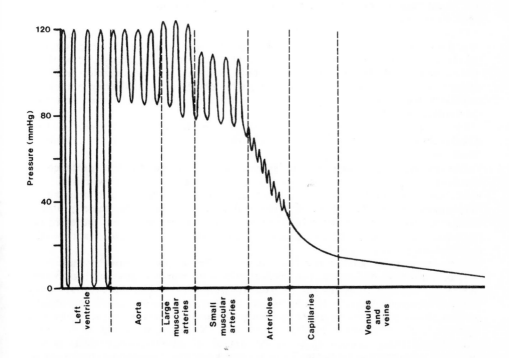

Figure 4.1. The changes in pressure which occur in the different types of vessels in the systemic circulation.

4.2.3 *Capillaries*

A smaller drop in pressure occurs across the capillaries. This is because these vessels offer less resistance to blood flow than the arterioles since their total cross-sectional area is greater. The walls of these short vessels, which are only about 5–10 μm in diameter, contain only a single layer of endothelial cells. Electron microscope studies have shown the existence of three types of capillary.

The most common type is the continuous or non-fenestrated capillary. These have no recognisable openings within the cells but there are spaces between the cells. Some of these spaces contain channels about 4 nm wide and these appear to be the routes by which fluid and water-soluble substances exchange with the interstitial fluid. In the brain, the junctions between the cells are tight and do not contain channels. Thus, these capillaries act as a barrier to the passage of many lipid-insoluble substances into the brain.

A second type, the fenestrated capillaries, occurs within organs which are concerned with filtration, secretion or absorption, such as the kidney, glands and intestine. These capillaries have openings within the cell walls whose function is probably to allow the rapid transfer of large amounts of fluid across the capillary walls.

The third type of capillary, the discontinuous capillary, is often termed a sinusoid. These capillaries have large gaps between the individual cells of the endothelium which allow the transfer of large molecules such as proteins as well as red blood cells. Sinusoids are found within the bone marrow, liver and spleen. It is not always possible to correlate the permeability of capillaries to different substances with the size of openings in the membrane which can be seen by means of the electron microscope.

Capillaries are the site at which the exchange of substances between the blood and tissues occurs and it is this exchange which is the ultimate function of the cardiovascular system. Four types of transport occur across the walls of the capillaries: diffusion, pinocytosis, bulk flow of fluid and carrier-mediated transport. The ease with which different molecules are transported across the capillary walls depends upon the properties of both the substance and that particular capillary.

Small lipid-soluble molecules such as carbon dioxide and oxygen diffuse freely through the endothelium of the capillaries down their concentration gradients.

The passage of lipid-insoluble substances is limited by the presence of openings, both within the cell walls and between the cells, which are of different sizes in the different types of capillaries. Pinocytosis may be of importance in the transport of large molecules, for example, some proteins, into the tissues. In the brain, carrier proteins are important in the selective transport of some substances, e.g. glucose and amino acids, across the capillaries.

The forces which govern the filtration and absorption of fluid by bulk flow across capillary walls are the hydrostatic and osmotic pressure gradients across the walls. Values for the hydrostatic pressures within the capillary vary depending upon the site of the vessel. In the glomerular capillaries of the kidney, mean capillary pressure is about 50 mmHg, whereas in the lungs and liver it is about 8 and 6 mmHg respectively. Hydrostatic pressures will also vary considerably depending upon the degree of constriction present in the pre- and post-capillary vessels. Typical values for the hydrostatic pressures in the capillaries can, however, be used to illustrate the forces governing the transfer of fluid across the capillaries.

In early studies of the pressure in a typical systemic capillary of the continuous type, as found in, for example, skeletal muscle, capillary pressure at the arteriolar end of the capillary was found to be about 32 mmHg and, at the venous end, about 15 mmHg. Thus, the mean capillary pressure was about 24 mmHg. Later experiments suggested that the hydrostatic pressure exerted by the interstitial fluid may be as much as 6 mmHg below atmospheric pressure and that the pressures within the capillaries were lower than first thought (25 mmHg at the arteriolar end and 10 mmHg at the venous end). Thus, the hydrostatic pressure gradient at the arteriolar end pushing fluid out is 31 mmHg and, at the venous end, 16 mmHg. These outward forces are opposed by the oncotic pressure which is the osmotic pressure exerted by the plasma proteins which, unlike the electrolytes, are not freely permeable through the membrane. Albumin is particularly important in this respect since it has a lower molecular weight than the globulins and is also present in a higher concentration in blood than are the globulins. Thus, the number of osmotically active molecules of albumin is far greater than that of the globulins. The osmotic pressure exerted by the plasma proteins (the oncotic pressure) is approximately 25 mmHg. This osmotic pressure tending to draw fluid into the capillaries will be offset to some degree by the osmotic pressure exerted by the proteins present in the interstitial fluid. The concentration of protein within the interstitial fluid will vary depending upon the type of capillary. In skeletal muscle, where the capillaries are of the continuous type, it is approximately 10–30 per cent of the plasma protein concentration. In the intestine, where there are fenestrated capillaries, it may be as high as 40–60 per cent of the plasma concentration and in the liver, where there are sinusoids, interstitial fluid protein concentration may be as much as 80–90 per cent of the plasma levels. Thus, the net osmotic force will vary from tissue to tissue.

The forces operating across a typical systemic capillary are shown in Figure 4.2. Values of 5 mmHg are assumed for the osmotic pressure exerted by the proteins in the interstitial fluid and 6 mmHg below atmospheric pressure for the interstitial hydrostatic pressure. At the arteriolar end of the capillary, the net outward hydrostatic pressure exceeds the net osmotic pressure, therefore, fluid will move from the capillary out into the interstitial space. At the venous end of the capillary, the net outward hydrostatic pressure is exceeded by the net osmotic pressure, therefore, fluid will be drawn back into the capillary. Most of the filtered fluid is reabsorbed but some enters the lymphatic system (see Section 4.4).

Changes in either the hydrostatic pressures or the oncotic pressures influence the transfer of fluid across the capillary. Disturbances in the normal equilibrium between these forces may result in the excessive filtration of fluid and its accumulation within the interstitial space (oedema).

The balance between the pressures within the pre-capillary and post-capillary vessels is important in determining the amount of fluid filtered. Capillary pressures may be increased by an increase in the central venous pressure. Changes in the degree of vasoconstriction in the two sets of vessels can also modify the amount of fluid filtered. For example, vasodilator metabolites produced by active tissues tend to act on the precapillary vessels increasing capillary pressures and thus increasing filtration, whereas sympathetic vasoconstrictor nerves act at both pre- and post-capillary sites and tend to reduce capillary pressures and thus increase reabsorption. Changes in the degree of constriction of different resistance vessels could result in some capillaries filtering and others reabsorbing along their length.

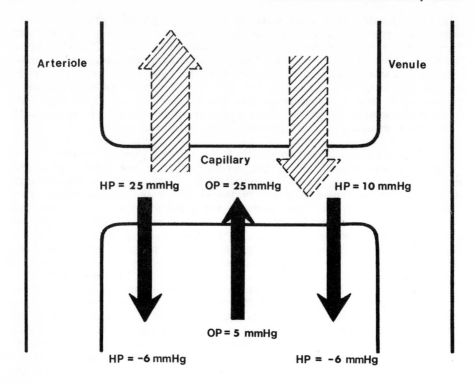

Interstitium

Figure 4.2. The forces operating across a typical systemic capillary due to differences in the hydrostatic pressures (HP) and oncotic pressure (OP). The large hatched arrows represent the net movement of fluid across the capillary walls.

Reductions in plasma protein concentration resulting, for example, from a decreased protein intake (as occurs in malnutrition) may also result in oedema.

This sequence of filtration at the arteriolar end of the capillary followed by absorption at the venous end along the length of the capillary is not found in all capillaries. In the pulmonary circulation, for example, capillary pressures are lower than oncotic pressures along the full length of the capillary and therefore there is absorption only along the length of the capillary. In the glomerular capillaries of the kidney, pressures are much higher than in most tissues and there is filtration along much of the length of the capillary. Because relatively large amounts of fluid, but not protein, leave the capillaries, the oncotic pressure rises along the length of the capillary and filtration ceases when the net hydrostatic and oncotic pressures are equal. Thus, in the glomerular capillaries, in contrast to the events occurring in capillaries in skeletal muscle, the hydrostatic pressures remain relatively constant but the oncotic pressure rises along the length of the capillary until equilibrium is reached.

Normally, at rest, only about a quarter of the capillaries will be perfused at any one time. In some vascular beds, e.g. skeletal muscle, even fewer capillaries are perfused at rest. Changes in the number of capillaries perfused will affect the surface area available for diffusion and the distance substances have to diffuse. It is now clear that, in most circulations, whether or not a particular capillary is perfused does not depend upon the active contraction of the precapillary vessels. Instead, passive factors are important, such as changes in the transmural pressure across the vessels or the plugging, and thus effective closure, of capillaries by blood cells.

4.2.4 *Venules and veins*
Pressure continues to drop across the venous side of the circulation. The venules leading from the capillaries contain a small amount of connective tissue and muscle which increases as the size of the vessels increases. These vessels are termed veins once their diameter exceeds 500 μm and, in these vessels, the endothelial lining may become folded to produce the venous

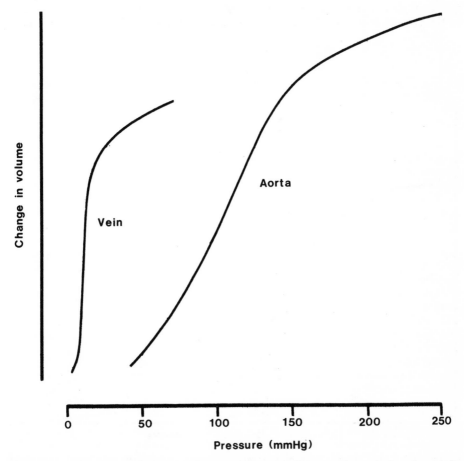

Figure 4.3. The relationship between the change in volume and the change in pressure (compliance) of a large vein and of the aorta.

valves. These valves are not present in all veins, but are present in the veins within the legs. The veins have thinner walls than the arteries but contain the same three basic layers, although the demarcation between the layers is less clear and there is more variation between veins from different regions. Veins are much more distensible than the small muscular arterioles and, thus, these vessels have a capacitance function rather than the resistance function of the arterioles.

The relationship between the change in volume within the vessel and the transmural pressure across the vessel for both a vein and a large elastic artery (like the aorta) is shown in Figure 4.3. Even though, at normal arterial pressures, the aorta is distensible, as the pressure increases, the vessel becomes more rigid. At normal venous pressures, veins are very much more distensible than even elastic arteries.

Veins are commonly semi-collapsed into an elliptical shape because their transmural pressures are low. As their transmural pressure increases, they become circular in cross-section and thus their resistance to flow decreases and their capacitance increases. Thus, much of the increase in capacitance which occurs when the transmural pressure rises from low values of about 6–9 cmH_2O is not a measure of the true distensibility of the veins but is due to the change in shape of the vessels. In recumbent man, about 60–70 per cent

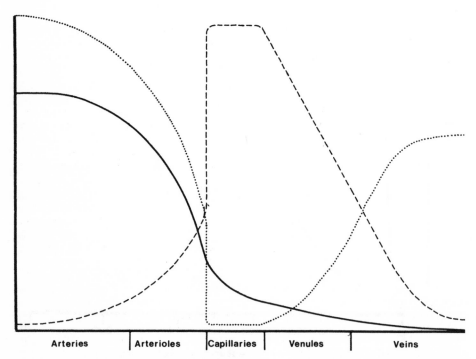

Figure 4.4. The changes in mean pressure (———), total cross-sectional area (---) and linear velocity of flow (......) which occur in the different vessels in the systemic circulation.

of the blood volume is found in the veins and venules, the vast majority of this capacitance function being provided by the small veins and the venules. Changes in the pressure within the venules and small veins are an important factor in determining the forces operating across the capillaries (see Section 4.2.3).

Thus, pressure drops across the systemic circulation, but, at the same time, there are important changes in the total cross-sectional area occupied by the different groups of vessels and in the average linear velocity of blood flow in the different vessels (see Figure 4.4). As the vessels branch, the total cross-sectional area increases from a value of about 4 cm^2 in the windkessel vessels to 2500–3000 cm^2 in the capillaries, reducing again through the venous side of the circulation. This increase in cross-sectional area will influence the velocity of blood flow so that this is slowest in the capillaries and at its maximum in the large elastic arteries.

4.3 Venous return

The mechanisms by which the output of the heart can be altered have been discussed in Section 3.2. However, other than on a beat-to-beat basis, cardiac output can only be maintained at any particular level if it is equalled by venous return. If blood vessels were rigid structures the driving force which determines venous return to the heart would be the pressure gradient between the left ventricle and the right atrium (the *vis a tergo*). However, since blood vessels are distensible, an increase in this pressure gradient will not necessarily increase the venous return.

Venous return is greatly influenced by the posture of the subject. When a subject stands, the transmural pressures of the veins above the heart fall. This tends to cause these veins to collapse. Conversely, below the heart, the transmural pressures increase, the veins distend and blood pools in the legs. When a man is standing motionless, the hydrostatic pressures recorded in all the vessels in the foot increase by about 85–100 mmHg compared to the values obtained in the supine position. The pressure gradients between the vessels remain the same. These high hydrostatic pressures in the capillaries would result in an increased filtration of fluid from the capillaries and the accumulation of fluid within the interstitial space. However, normally, there are movements of the legs, and even slight leg movements will exert pressure on the veins and push the columns of blood towards the heart and the presence of valves in the leg veins will prevent backflow of blood. Increasing the force and frequency of muscle contractions will result in an increase in venous return. These movements will dramatically reduce the venous pressures recorded at the feet (see Figure 4.5).

Changes in central venous pressure also affect venous return. During inspiration, central venous pressure is reduced and this will increase the pressure gradient along which blood flows from the periphery to the right atrium, thus increasing venous return. The suction effects exerted by the ventricles both when they contract and when they relax (*vis a fronte*), may also influence venous return but these effects are small in man. The *vis a fronte* is more important in small, rapidly-contracting hearts.

Venous return can also be influenced by the action of the sympathetic constrictor fibres which innervate the veins and venules. This vasocontrictor action is important when the veins are well-filled and distended, as occurs in the leg veins in the erect posture. When the transmural pressure is low and the veins are semi-collapsed, the action of vasoconstrictor fibres may result in an

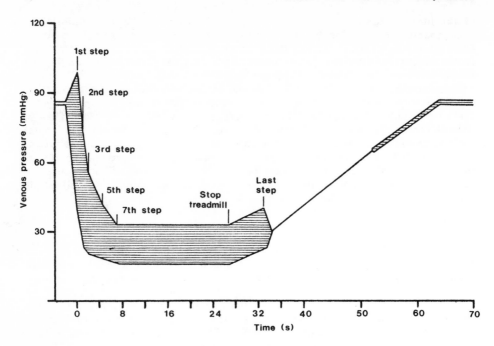

Figure 4.5. Average changes in venous pressure, recorded at the ankle, in ten subjects, produced by walking on a treadmill (From Pollack & Wood, 1949).

increase in capacitance by making the vessels more circular in shape even though their circumference is decreased.

4.4 The lymphatic system

The primary function of the lymphatic system is to provide a system for the drainage of excess fluid, protein, lipids and foreign materials from the interstitial spaces into the blood. Thus, it supplements the drainage function of the venous system.

The lymphatic capillaries are blind-ending sacs whose walls are composed of a single layer of endothelial cells. These capillaries are distributed freely throughout the tissues of the body. Thus, in these two respects, they resemble the capillaries of the systemic circulation. However, unlike the systemic capillaries, the lymphatic capillaries are freely permeable to proteins and other large molecules. Thus dying blood cells, bacteria and foreign particles will enter the lymphatics. After a meal, lipid-containing chylomicra enter the lymphatics from the intestine, giving the lymph its characteristic milky appearance.

These lymphatic capillaries join to form lymphatic vessels which, like the veins, have an increasing proportion of elastic tissue and muscle in their walls as they increase in size. Like the veins, their endothelium is also folded to form valves which allow only unidirectional flow towards the central veins. Lymph glands are found distributed along the larger lymphatic vessels. The lymphatic vessels subdivide into a number of smaller vessels which open into the sinuses of the glands, allowing substances such as lymphocytes and γ-globulins to enter the lymphatic system. These smaller vessels then join up again to form large vessels. The final channels, the right and left thoracic ducts, empty into the subclavian veins.

Macromolecules which enter the lymphatic vessels can only escape from the system by entering the bloodstream. However, molecules of molecular weight below 5000 can readily escape from the lymphatic system. The mechanisms which allow large molecules to enter the lymphatic vessels but prevent them from leaving are not clear. Some authorities believe that macromolecules enter the lymphatic system by pinocytosis, whereas others favour the existence of gaps between the cells of the endothelial layer. Once in the capillaries, the molecules are propelled along the lymphatic system and, in the larger vessels, retrograde flow is prevented by the valves in the endothelium. The walls of the larger lymphatic vessels are not permeable to macromolecules and thus the molecules are unable to leave the lymphatic system until the lymph drains into the large veins.

The composition of lymph is similar to that of plasma except that, on average, the protein concentration is lower. The protein concentration in the lymph varies from region to region; in the liver it is about 6 $g \cdot l^{-1}$ whereas, at rest, in the lymph vessels of the leg it is only about 1–2 $g \cdot l^{-1}$. Pressure within the lymphatics is similar to that of the interstitial fluid and fluctuates between about -3 mmHg and +5mmHg relative to atmospheric pressure.

The flow of lymph in man is relatively sluggish, only about 2–4 litres per day, which is approximately equal to the plasma volume. The flow of the lymph is increased by muscular exercise, by massage, if the venous pressure is raised or if there is vasodilatation or an increase in the permeability of the systemic capillaries. In glandular tissue, lymph flow is increased when the gland is secreting.

Local blockage of lymph vessels will result in the accumulation of protein within the interstitial space and thus lead to oedema (see Section 4.2.3).

Further reading

Bundgaard, M. (1980). Transport pathways in capillaries — in search of pores. *Ann. Rev. Physiol.* **42**, 325—36.

Burton, A.C. (1969). *Physiology and Biophysics of the Circulation.* Year Book Medical Publishers: Chicago.

Gore, R.W. & McDonagh, P.F. (1980). Fluid exchange across single capillaries. *Ann. Rev. Physiol.* **42**, 337—57.

Mayersen, H.S. (1966). The physiologic importance of lymph. In: *Handbook of Physiology, Section 2, Circulation,* Volume II, *Vascular Smooth Muscle,* pp. 1035—73. American Physiological Society: Bethesda.

Rothe, C.F. (1983). Venous system: physiology of the capacitance vessels. In: *Handbook of Physiology, Section 2, The Cardiovascular System,* Volume III, Part 1, pp. 397—452. American Physiological Society; Bethesda.

5

MECHANISMS REGULATING BLOOD FLOW TO DIFFERENT REGIONS

In Chapter 4, I described the different types of vessels in the circulation and showed that, in the systemic circulation, the main resistance to blood flow was exerted by the arterioles. In this chapter, I shall discuss the mechanisms whereby the amount of blood flowing to different organs and tissues can be altered. These changes in the distribution of the blood flow are brought about largely by changing the resistance to blood flow. From the Hagen—Poiseuille equation (see Section 1.3.1.1), the major determinant of resistance is the radius of the blood vessels. Thus, when we are looking at the mechanisms which are responsible for diverting flow from one part of the circulation to another, what we are really looking at are the mechanisms which alter the radius of the arterioles in the different circulations.

5.1 Distribution of cardiac output

Many measurements have been made of the distribution of the cardiac output at rest. An example of results from such a study is shown in Table 5.1. The

Table 5.1. Table to show the distribution of cardiac output to some of the major tissues and organs of the body at rest.

Organ or Tissue	Percentage of cardiac output
Kidney	23
Central nervous system	15
Skeletal muscle	15
Gastro-intestinal tract	14
Liver (via hepatic artery)	10
Heart	4
Skin	4

largest proportion (about a quarter) of the cardiac output goes to the kidneys. In addition, the central nervous system, skeletal muscle, gastro-intestinal tract and liver each receive a significant proportion (10–15 per cent) of the cardiac output. A smaller proportion of the cardiac output is distributed to the heart and skin. Such an analysis of the overall distribution of cardiac output at rest and the way in which this distribution alters in different circumstances is a useful aid to our understanding of how the cardiovascular system functions as a whole. However, if we want to compare blood flow in different circulations under differing circumstances, a more useful approach is to express blood flow in terms of flow per 100 g of tissue. This convention will be adopted for the rest of this chapter.

If we now look at the values for blood flows to different areas of the body, expressed as $ml \cdot min^{-1} \cdot 100g$ of tissue^{-1} in a resting subject at a comfortable temperature (see Table 5.2), we can see which parts of the body receive a high resting blood flow and which receive a lower resting blood flow. For a naked man the comfortable enviromental temperature is about 27 °C but this will obviously be less if he is clothed. At rest, the kidney receives an enormous blood flow. Blood flow to the heart and brain is high too, but blood flow to skeletal muscle at rest is very low.

The degree by which blood flow to different regions can change also varies very much between regions; for example, blood flow to the kidney and brain remains relatively constant whereas blood flow to the heart, gastro-intestinal tract and skeletal muscle varies over a large range (see Chapter 6 for a further discussion of the different regional circulations). It is useful here to divide the circulations into two groups: the high-priority circulations and the low-priority circulations. The high-priority circulations are the circulations to the brain, the heart and, to a lesser extent, the kidney. Blood flow to these circulations must be maintained as a priority. Thus, if cardiac output is reduced, for example, following a haemorrhage, the maintenance of blood

Table 5.2. Table to show blood flow (expressed as $ml \cdot min^{-1} \cdot 100g^{-1}$) to different organs and tissues in man at rest at a comfortable environmental temperature.

Organ or Tissue	Blood flow $ml \cdot min^{-1} \cdot 100g^{-1}$
Kidney	400
Heart	60–80
Central nervous system	50–60
Gastro–intestinal tract	15–40
Skin	20
Skeletal muscle	2–5

flow to the brain and the heart and then to the kidney are given the highest priority. Under such a stress, the blood flow to the low-priority circulations, for example skeletal muscle, skin and the gastro-intestinal tract, will be severely reduced. This division between high- and low-priority circulations is not, however, fixed, and under some circumstances the maintenance of blood flow to what is normally a low-priority circulation, for example, the skin, may become paramount. This will occur in severe heat stress where blood flow to the skin is increased in order to lose heat from the body.

What, then, are the mechanisms which regulate the diameter of the arterioles and hence the blood flow to the different regions? These mechanisms can be readily divided into two groups: firstly, those which act locally in response to a local stimulus and, secondly, those mechanisms which are controlled from a distance via changes in the activity of nerves and the release of hormones from distant sites. Actions mediated via nervous and hormonal mechanisms can be controlled from within the central nervous system so that an integrated response occurs, appropriate to the particular circumstance. For example, during exercise, blood flow needs to be diverted away from the gastro-intestinal tract to the exercising muscle, whereas, when environmental temperature is high, blood needs to be directed towards the skin (see Chapter 9 for further discussion of these changes).

5.2 Effects of local factors on blood flow

In the absence of stimulation by vasoconstrictor hormones or nerves, most blood vessels are electrically and mechanically quiescent. However, the exceptions to this are the small arterioles. These vessels are capable of constricting, even when all external influences have been removed. This is termed their myogenic activity. It is caused by the instability of the resting membrane potential in the smooth muscle. Spontaneous depolarisation of the membrane will ultimately lead to a contraction of the smooth muscle. This depolarisation spreads from one cell to another, since in smooth muscle, as in cardiac muscle, there are areas of low resistance between the muscle cells. Conduction is much better around the vessel than along it. The effects remain localised. Each arteriole is generally capable of contracting independently of other arterioles.

This resting myogenic activity is enhanced by distending the vessels. *In vivo* this will occur as a result of an increase in intravascular or transmural pressures. Thus, distension of a vessel will result in vasoconstriction. Myogenic activity can also be modified by nerves and hormones, as will be discussed later (see Section 5.3 & 5.4).

The level of myogenic activity varies very much between vessels from different parts of the body. In general, it is highest in those blood vessels in which the blood flow changes greatly, for example, arterioles in skeletal muscle and salivary glands. Myogenic activity is absent or very low in most veins. However, in the portal and anterior mesenteric veins and in some of the medium and large lymph vessels both spontaneous changes in electrical activity and spontaneous contractions are found.

A number of factors, mainly the breakdown products of metabolism, also act locally to alter the radius of the blood vessels. These mainly act on the pre-capillary resistance vessels rather than the post-capillary sites. Many factors will result in a vasodilatation of the arterioles. These include hypoxia, an increase in the pCO_2 or the concentration of hydrogen ions, potassium ions or lactate, the presence of breakdown products of ATP (such as adenosine) and an increase in the number of osmotically active particles in the vessel (hyperosmolality). Much attention was paid in the past to finding the 'key metabolite', with no success. It appears that, although many vasodilator substances have been found, their importance varies in different circulations. For example, vasodilatation in coronary blood vessels seems to be controlled by hypoxia, whereas, in the brain, the concentration of hydrogen ions in the fluid surrounding the vessels seems to be of more importance.

Vasodilator substances act by relaxing the vessel walls. Hydrogen ions are thought to exert their effects by competing for, and partially blocking, sodium and calcium channels in the cell membrane, thus reducing the influx of these ions and hyperpolarising the cell membrane. A given decrease in blood pH produced by an increase in CO_2 results in a greater relaxation of arteries than the same change produced by non-respiratory acids. This is because CO_2 readily enters the cell and will increase intracellular acidity. Changes in the intracellular acidity probably directly affect the contractile proteins. There are many possible ways in which hypoxia could produce its relaxant effects. For example it might act by reducing ATP levels below the optimal level for contraction or via some intermediary.

The importance of these local metabolites can be readily demonstrated in man. If a cuff is inflated around the upper arm so that the pressure in the cuff exceeds the systolic blood pressure, then blood flow to that arm will be stopped. During the period of this occlusion, metabolism in the tissues of the arm will continue and therefore, there will be an accumulation of vasodilator metabolites in the arm and the arterioles will dilate. When the occluding cuff is removed and blood flow to the arm is re-established, the level of blood flow will be very much greater than it was at rest. This increase in blood flow can be measured using a plethysmograph (see Section 10.2.6.4) but can also be shown more simply by observing the change in skin colour. After removal of the cuff the arm is red in colour and feels warm, indicating an increased blood flow. This increase in blood flow, following a period of restricted blood flow, is termed reactive hyperaemia. In fact, reactive hyperaemia is often unintentionally demonstrated by students learning to measure blood pressure using such a cuff.

Thus, if we have removed all the external influences from the blood vessel, the radius of the vessel is determined by the balance between the myogenic activity of the smooth muscle, which is tending to constrict the vessel and which will be increased if the vessel is distended, and the effects of the locally-released metabolites which will cause vasodilatation of the vessel. These local factors are important, not only in contributing towards the redistribution of blood flow, but also in maintaining blood flow and capillary pressure relatively constant in the face of changes in perfusion pressure.

In a rigid tube or a piece of dead tissue, if the perfusion pressure is increased, this will lead to an increase in the flow. However, in many vessels of the body, blood flow can remain relatively constant in spite of changes in perfusion pressure. This phenomenon is known as autoregulation and is particularly marked in the blood vessels of the kidney (see Figure 5.1). The maintenance of a constant blood flow in the face of a rise in perfusion pressure must mean that the resistance has increased and constant blood flow in the face of a fall in perfusion pressure must mean that the resistance has decreased. These changes in resistance to flow in the vessels are brought about by local effects on the vessels.

Let us first look at the effect of a rise in perfusion pressure to a vessel, brought about by an increase in the arterial blood pressure. This will have two effects, both of which will increase the amount of vasoconstriction of the

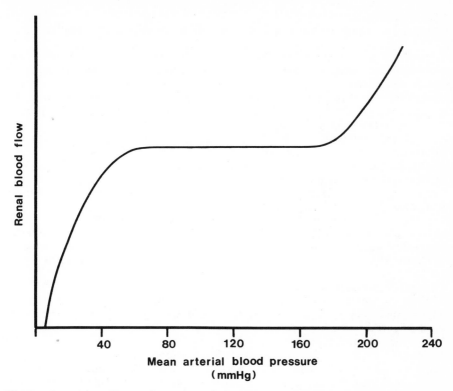

Figure 5.1. The effect of changes in mean arterial blood pressure on renal blood flow.

vessel. Firstly, the increase in pressure will distend the vessel and thus increase its myogenic activity. Secondly, the increase in pressure will initially increase blood flow and thus wash out the vasodilator metabolites. Thus, the increase in perfusion pressure will be balanced by an increase in the resistance to blood flow, so blood flow will remain relatively constant. In the opposite example, where blood pressure falls, this will lead to a reduction in the myogenic activity of the vessel and an accumulation of vasodilator metabolites. The result will be vasodilatation and a fall in the resistance to blood flow. Consequently, the change in resistance will oppose the change in pressure and, as a result, blood flow will be maintained relatively constant.

This autoregulation is important for two reasons: firstly, it allows the maintenance of a constant flow of blood, and thus a constant supply of oxygen and nutrients, to a tissue in the face of changing levels of arterial blood pressure; secondly, these local adjustments in the diameter of the vessels are important in regulating capillary pressure, and, thus (as was discussed in Section 4.2.3), in regulating tissue fluid volume. In studies on skeletal muscle capillaries, it was found that changing the arterial pressure through a range of 30 to 170 mmHg changed capillary pressure by only about 2 mmHg either side of the normal value. However, in the absence of local regulatory mechanisms, changes in the pressure over this range would be expected to alter capillary pressure by about 10 mmHg either side of normal values, resulting in a net movement of fluid of between 30 and 75 $ml \cdot min^{-1}$ for the whole muscle mass.

Changes in venous pressure will also result in an increase in the myogenic activity in the pre-capillary vessels. Under these circumstances, the maintenance of constant capillary pressures takes precedence over the maintenance of constant flow. When venous pressures increase, there is an increase in the myogenic activity of the pre-capillary resistance vessels and vasoconstriction will tend to reduce blood flow. Whether or not this vasoconstriction will be seen depends on the balance between the myogenic activity and the action of the vasodilator metabolites. If blood flow is in excess of the metabolic needs of the tissue then the myogenic activity will predominate and blood flow will decrease. However, if blood flow is low initially, and is only adequate to meet the nutritional needs of the tissue, then a vasoconstriction will not be seen.

Changes in myogenic activity may be important during postural changes. When changing from the recumbent to the upright position, hydrostatic pressures in the legs will increase (see Section 1.3). It may be that the resultant increase in myogenic activity, which itself will result in a lowering of capillary pressures in the legs, may prevent the filtration of an excess of fluid from the capillaries and, thus, prevent the formation of oedema in the legs.

Changes in pressure outside the vessel, by altering transmural pressures, may also alter myogenic activity. These changes in extravascular pressure will, for example, occur in skeletal or cardiac muscle during the transition between rest and contraction.

Thus, the maintenance of a constant capillary pressure, as well as the maintenance of a constant blood flow, is an important function of the local regulatory adjustments considered above. It seems that factors which act quickly to change myogenic activity primarily control capillary pressures and, although these changes in myogenic activity may influence blood flow, this is primarily controlled at a local level by the action of the vasodilator metabolites.

Autoregulation is most pronounced in the renal circulation and is particularly important in the kidney, since a steady capillary pressure and blood flow are necessary for filtration and reabsorption. However, renal blood vessels show very little myogenic activity, so the mechanisms described above cannot explain the very large degree of autoregulation exerted by the kidney (see Section 6.6).

In addition to the effects of changes in myogenic activity and the presence of vasodilator substances on the pre-capillary resistance vessels, there are also a number of vasoactive substances which may be released locally and act locally. One example of such a substance is histamine, a powerful vasodilator of small arteries and arterioles. The kinins, of which bradykinin is the best known, are also powerful vasodilator agents on these vessels. Prostaglandins, too, may be released locally. Different prostaglandins have different actions in different parts of the circulation. The possible role of kinins and prostaglandins in the control of the circulation remains controversial at present, but they have been implicated in a number of responses, particularly in the kidney. For example, by producing a vasodilatation of renal blood vessels, prostaglandins may be responsible for maintaining renal blood flow during anaesthesia. Both histamine and bradykinin, although they dilate small arteries, constrict large arteries. However, their dilator effects on the small vessels, which are the major site of resistance, are likely to be of greater physiological significance than their effects on the large vessels.

Injury to blood vessels can also produce profound effects. The direct response to injury of a blood vessel is a local vasoconstriction which is thought to be due in large part to depolarisation conducted from one cell to another around the artery wall. The more extensive contractions caused by an extensive crushing or tearing injury, involving a large part of the vessel, are thought to be due to an increased influx of extracellular calcium ions. If a blood clot is formed 5-hydroxy-tryptamine (5-HT or serotonin), is released from the platelets. This substance is a very powerful vasoconstrictor agent.

Changes in temperature can also directly affect blood vessels. Cooling the skin of the limbs to between 12°C and 25°C produces a reduction in blood flow which is partly attributable to a direct effect on the blood vessels, and partly due to the increased activity of sympathetic vasoconstrictor fibres (see Section 5.3). The direct effects are thought to result from a slowing of the electrogenic sodium—potassium pump and a subsequent depolarisation of the membrane. Contraction in the smooth muscle is presumably brought about by the entry of calcium ions into the cells. Cooling will also reduce the removal of noradrenaline after its release from nerve terminals.

In contrast, cooling to below 12°C will also act locally on blood vessels but will result in a failure of both their electrical and mechanical activity. The resultant paralysis of the smooth muscle will cause the vessel to dilate. Under these conditions, the effects of nerves on the smooth muscle will also be inhibited. This cold vasodilatation explains the bright red colour of the skin when immersed in very cold water. This dilatation is delayed in onset, is very localised, and is intermittent, being interrupted every few minutes by waves of constriction which are separated by waves of vasodilatation (see Figure 5.2). This phenomenon is known as 'hunting'. The initial vasoconstriction of the blood vessels results in a fall in temperature within the blood vessel and thus paralysis of the smooth muscle and vasodilatation. The blood flowing through the area will be warm and thus allows the vessel to contract again.

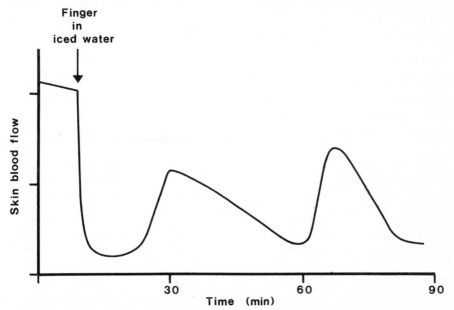

Figure 5.2. The effect of immersion of a finger in iced water on blood flow to the skin.

5.3 Effects of nerves on blood flow

In addition to all the effects at a local level, the radius of blood vessels can be greatly altered by nerves and hormones. Changes in the activity of these nerves is induced in the central nervous system (see Section 8.1), far away from the sites of the vessels. The release of some of the hormones is also controlled from the central nervous system. This control by nerves and hormones can, therefore, be thought of as the long-distance rather than the local control mechanism. Effects mediated by nervous mechanisms have the additional advantage that they can be produced very quickly.

Let us deal first with the influence of nerves on blood vessels. There are different groups of nerves which produce either vasoconstriction or vasodilatation of blood vessels. The vasoconstrictor fibres are part of the sympathetic nervous system. This is the most important nervous mechanism controlling blood flow in most circulations. The distribution of these sympathetic nerves to blood vessels is widespread. They innervate large and small arteries, arterioles and veins. However, the density of innervation of different blood vessels does vary between circulations. For example, the blood vessels in the skin receive a dense innervation, whereas blood vessels in the brain receive a much more sparse innervation from the sympathetic vasoconstrictor fibres.

In small arteries, the nerves are generally confined to the tunica adventitia, the outermost layer of the blood vessel wall, whereas in large arteries, such as the carotid artery, the outer half of the smooth muscle also receives a dense innervation of vasoconstrictor fibres. The inner muscle of both the large and small arteries in the systemic circulation is free of adrenergic or any other nerves. Exceptions to this are the terminal parts of the pulmonary arterioles in which the nerves may penetrate the entire muscle coat. In veins too, the nerves often penetrate the entire muscle coat. The reason nerves are absent from the inner parts of the vessel wall appears to be that they cannot penetrate the region of high pressure in the tissue near the lumen of the vessel. Pressure within the vessel wall will vary from mean arterial pressure (approximately 100 mmHg) near the lumen to atmospheric pressure in the outer part of the wall. Artificially raising the pressure within the whole of the vessel wall by placing a clip around the artery results in a degeneration of adrenergic nerve fibres from the entire vessel wall. The ability of nerve fibres to penetrate the entire muscular wall of pulmonary arterioles and of veins can, therefore, readily be explained in terms of the lower pressures within these vessels and, thus, the lower pressure gradients within the vessel walls.

This difference in the innervation of the outer and inner muscle layers is reflected in the different sensitivity of these two layers to noradrenaline. The inner layer is 10 to 100 times more sensitive to low concentrations of noradrenaline than is the outer layer and this difference is a real difference in the sensitivity of the two regions and is not solely due to the reuptake of noradrenaline into the nerve terminals situated in the outermost layer. Similar differences in the sensitivity of the inner and outer layers are found in response to histamine, angiotensin and adrenaline, none of which are taken up by nerve terminals in appreciable amounts.

Even though the difference in sensitivity between outer and inner layers of the smooth muscle is real, there is evidence that it is imposed upon the smooth muscle by its nerve supply. If a blood vessel is denervated, after a period of 10 to 42 days, these differences in sensitivity are greatly reduced.

Thus, catecholamines circulating in the blood act by causing the inner layer of smooth muscle to contract. The less sensitive outer layer of muscle requires the high concentrations of noradrenaline which are produced at adrenergic nerve endings to produce contraction. At high rates of sympathetic discharge, enough noradrenaline probably diffuses through the vessel wall to cause the inner layer of smooth muscle also to contract.

As yet, no such differences in the sensitivity of the inner and outer layers of the muscle to vasodilator substances, which are released by tissues outside the blood vessels, have been established. However, preliminary studies on coronary vessels, which receive an innervation from vasodilator nerves, suggest that there may be such differences in these vessels.

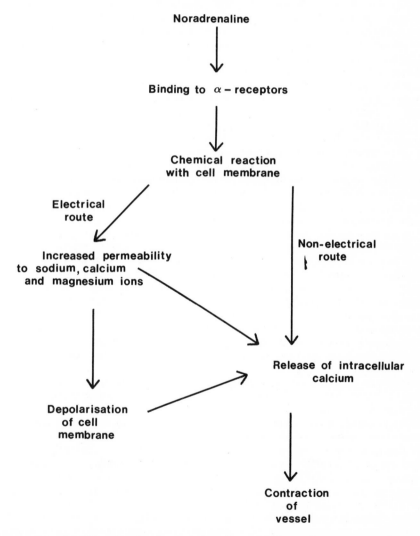

Figure 5.3. Possible mechanisms whereby noradrenaline can produce the release of intracellular calcium and, thus, constriction of a blood vessel.

Noradrenaline acts to constrict blood vessels by both an electrical and a non-electrical route (see Figure 5.3). The first stage is the binding of noradrenaline to α-receptors, followed by a chemical reaction with the cell membrane. In the case of low concentrations of circulating noradrenaline, this is often followed by a single spike and then a prolonged depolarisation. However, activation of the sympathetic nerve supply to an artery produces a series of brief irregular spike discharges. These spikes represent a rapid depolarisation of the membrane. This is caused by an increase in the permeability of the membrane to sodium and calcium ions and the subsequent entry of sodium and calcium ions down their electrochemical gradients. The presence of sodium ions seems to be necessary for an action potential to occur, calcium and magnesium ions being important in stabilising the membrane. The more sustained depolarisation is due to the opening of slow inward channels which allow calcium and magnesium ions to enter the cell. Repolarisation is due to the inactivation of the sodium and calcium channels and to an increase in the permeability of the cell membrane to potassium ions and may also involve chloride ions. These ionic changes differ in detail from the ionic changes underlying the action potential in cardiac muscle (see Section 2.4), but in principle are similar. Each spike represents the discharge from a particular group of smooth muscle cells. This asynchronous vasoconstrictor nerve activity results in a sustained contraction of the vessel wall rather than intermittent contractions of the vessel.

In the presence of anoxia, noradrenaline produces an initial discharge followed by a train of further discharges which result in a series of contractions. It has been suggested that these repetitive contractions might be the way in which the artery clears itself of obstructions to its lumen.

The calcium ions which enter the cells during the action potentials probably trigger the release of more calcium from stores as occurs in cardiac muscle (see Section 2.6). Thus, part of the mechanical response of the arteries to noradrenaline is brought about through a depolarisation. However, noradrenaline also acts directly to cause mechanical changes. Brief exposures to high concentrations of noradrenaline produce mechanical effects via changes in electrical activity, whereas the more prolonged action of low concentrations of noradrenaline is brought about by non-electrical means. Noradrenaline may cause contraction by non-electrical means by causing the release of calcium ions from stores without the initial entry of calcium ions during depolarisation. Noradrenaline could also increase the sensitivity of the contractile proteins to calcium without increasing the intracellular calcium levels.

Sympathetic vasoconstrictor nerves are tonically active, that is, even in a resting subject they are discharging. Early studies on anaesthetised animals suggested that the tonic rate of discharge of these nerves was between one and two impulses every second. However, recordings in conscious man of the sympathetic discharge to blood vessels suggests that, although tonically active, these fibres are discharging very much more slowly than originally thought — a few impulses every minute rather than every second. The discharge in individual sympathetic nerve fibres is normally irregular, although a small number of fibres do show a rhythm in phase with the heart beat or respiration. However, when recordings are made from groups of fibres within a sympathetic nerve, there is a pronounced cardiovascular rhythm to their firing. Thus, in some way, the discharge of individual fibres must be synchronised to produce the rhythm. This may occur within the brain or at the sympathetic ganglia.

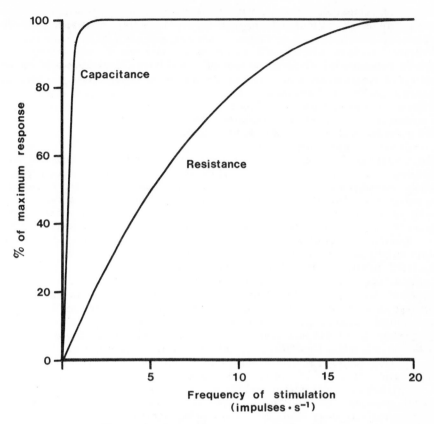

Figure 5.4. The effect of stimulating the sympathetic nerves to the blood vessels on the resistance and capacitance vessels in the systemic circulation.

This tonic activity is of physiological importance because it means that withdrawal of tonic vasoconstrictor activity will result in a vasodilatation of blood vessels and a subsequent increase in blood flow. The effect of removing the influence of the sympathetic nerves can be demonstated in the skeletal muscle circulation. At rest, blood flow to the skeletal muscle is about 2–5 $ml \cdot min^{-1} \cdot 100g^{-1}$. As a result of sectioning the sympathetic nerves to the blood vessels, blood flow will increase to approximately 6-9 $ml \cdot min^{-1} \cdot 100g^{-1}$.

Changes in the discharge of these sympathetic vasoconstrictor fibres will influence the radius of both resistance and capacitance vessels, that is, both arterioles and veins. Several studies have been carried out to show the relative importance of the effects of the sympathetic nerves on resistance and capacitance. An example of such a study is shown in Figure 5.4. It can be seen that the effects on capacitance occur at the lower range of frequencies of sympathetic stimulation — the maximal effects on the veins being produced at frequencies of stimulation of between one and two impulses per second. In contrast, the effects on resistance occur over a much larger range of frequencies, maximal effects being produced at frequencies of stimulation of about 15–20 impulses per second. In absolute terms, the maximal effects on resistance are much greater than those on capacitance.

Thus, the sympathetic nerves, with their widespread distribution to blood vessels, can have actions which will affect both the resistance and the capacitance vessels of the circulation. Their normal tonic activity means that withdrawal of their activity will result in a dilatation of both arteries and veins. In contrast, the different groups of vasodilator fibres have a much less widespread distribution and normally do not show tonic activity. There are four main groups of vasodilator fibres:

(1) Parasympathetic vasodilator fibres
(2) Sympathetic cholinergic vasodilator fibres
(3) Purinergic vasodilator fibres which release ATP
(4) Peptidergic vasodilator fibres.

The parasympathetic nerves release acetylcholine at their endings and have a limited distribution in the body. They innervate blood vessels supplying erectile tissues. Thus, it is increases in their discharge which are responsible for erection of the penis, clitoris and nipples. They also innervate blood vessels in a number of glands, such as salivary glands, and innervate the vessels in the gastro-intestinal tract. Within the glands, although there are some specific vasodilator fibres, much of the vasodilatation is due to the parasympathetic nerves releasing vasoactive substances such as vasoactive inhibitory peptide (VIP). Thus, much of the vasodilatation found during increased vagal activity is secondary to the production of vasodilator substances. Similarly, within, for example, the intestine, an increased vagal discharge is associated with an increased motility and secretion — and the formation of vasodilator substances within the intestine (see Section 6.7). The parasympathetic nerves also innervate the blood vessels in the brain and heart but the physiological significance of this innervation is not known.

In addition to the parasympathetic cholinergic nerves, there are also some sympathetic nerves which release acetylcholine at their endings. These are termed sympathetic cholinergic nerves and innervate the blood vessels within skeletal muscle. The functional significance of these nerves has been demonstrated in dogs and cats but their significance in man remains uncertain. In animals these nerves are important in producing the vasodilatation of blood vessels in skeletal muscle which is seen as part of the defence reaction (see Section 8.1). This is the classical alerting reaction seen in animals in response to the sight, sound or smell of a dangerous stimulus. Activation of these nerves is produced by stimulation within the area of the hypothalamus which is responsible for the initiation of the defence reaction. Whether or not activation of these nerves occurs in man as part of an alerting response or in anticipation of exercise remains a subject of speculation. There is evidence that, in man, part of the vasodilatation which occurs in skeletal muscle during stress (such as produced by mental arithmetic or alarming sounds) may be blocked by giving atropine. This suggests that the sympathetic cholinergic nerves to blood vessels in skeletal muscle may be important under these circumstances. This vasodilatation may be important in mediating the fainting, which can occur during emotional stress.

Research has shown that, in the systemic circulation, an intact endothelial layer of cells is necessary for acetylcholine to have its relaxant effects on blood vessels. It has been suggested that acetylcholine binds to receptors on the endothelium and causes the release of an unknown vasoactive mediator, possibly a prostaglandin, which produces relaxation of the smooth muscle and, therefore, vasodilatation.

In the pulmonary circulation, both acetylcholine and bradykinin require an intact endothelial layer in order to exert their vasodilator effects on blood vessels. When the endothelial layer of the blood vessels is damaged, these substances produce a contraction rather than a relaxation of the smooth muscle. This observation may be of clinical significance as it may explain why patients with pulmonary disease do not always respond to therapy with vasodilator drugs. In some of these patients, the pulmonary disease may have damaged the endothelial lining of the blood vessels.

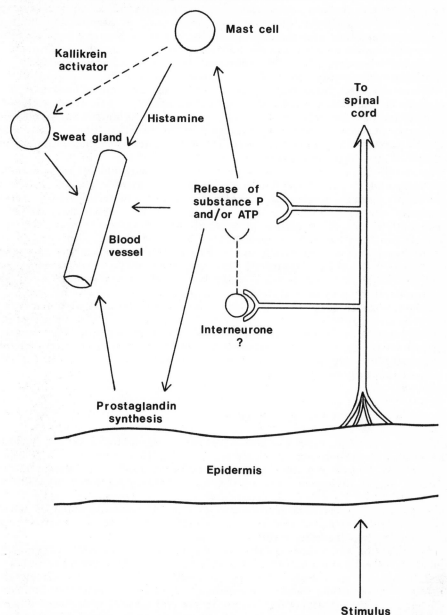

Figure 5.5. Possible mechanisms whereby stimulation of a sensory nerve might produce vasodilatation of a blood vessel.

The possible role of the remaining two groups of vasodilator nerves, the purinergic fibres and peptidergic fibres, is even more speculative. Purinergic nerves are thought to be involved in mediating the dilatation of the arterioles in the skin (the flare of the triple response - see Section 6.5) which occurs as a result of injury to the skin. When the skin is scratched, receptors at the point of injury are stimulated and action potentials travel up the sensory nerves through the dorsal roots into the spinal cord. It has been postulated that action potentials also travel antidromically down a branch of the sensory nerve and, either directly or via an interneurone, cause the release of a transmitter (possibly ATP or substance P) and subsequently lead to vasodilatation. At least part of this vasodilatation may be mediated via histamine released from mast cells, by ATP or by prostaglandins whose synthesis is induced by ATP. Kinins, activated by a kallikrein activator released by the mast cells, may also be involved (see Figure 5.5). A role for purinergic nerves has also been suggested in many other tissues, including skeletal muscle, lung and the gastro-intestinal tract, but the evidence in support of this suggestion is slim.

Peptidergic fibres have been identified associated with blood vessels both in the brain and in peripheral tissues, including the gastro-intestinal tract and the heart. A large number of peptides have been identified within nerve terminals but the role of these nerves has not, as yet, been clearly defined. The peptides are often found in association with other transmitters; for example, in the brain, neuropeptide Y (NPY) is found associated with noradrenergic nerve fibres and, in the gastro-intestinal tract, VIP is found associated with both sympathetic and parasympathetic nerves. Thus, in addition to any direct (mainly vasodilator) effects, they may have an important role to play in modulating the actions of the autonomic nerves.

Peptides released from nerve terminals, particularly VIP and NPY, may play a role in the regulation of cerebral blood flow. Both are found in the brain and VIP has been shown to produce vasodilatation of cerebral blood vessels, whereas NPY constricts these vessels. It has, therefore, been suggested that the release of NPY may be responsible for the cerebral vasospasm which follows subarachnoid haemorrhage in man.

5.4 Effects of hormones on blood flow

Circulating catecholamines can also affect the radius of blood vessels. In man, the adrenal medulla produces mainly adrenaline, although some noradrenaline is produced. In cats and dogs, a mixture of noradrenaline and adrenaline is secreted, and in diving animals and the human fetus, mainly noradrenaline is produced.

Noradrenaline acts via α receptors to produce a vasoconstriction of blood vessels. Circulating noradrenaline tends to affect the inner layer of smooth muscle more than the outer layers.

The actions of adrenaline on blood vessels are more complex. Adrenaline can act via α receptors to produce vasoconstriction or via β receptors to produce vasodilatation. The overall effect of adrenaline in a particular circulation will depend upon the relative numbers of α and β receptors and the concentration of circulating adrenaline. In skeletal muscle, where both α and β receptors are present in the blood vessels, adrenaline will produce vasodilatation at low doses and vasoconstriction at higher doses. This vasodilatation may be of physiological significance in situations, such as exercise, where blood flow through skeletal muscle needs to be increased. In other circulations, such as the heart, the β effects predominate at all concentrations of adrenaline and, thus, adrenaline always results in a vasodilatation of coronary blood vessels. In other circulations, for example, the skin, adrenaline results in a vasoconstriction which is mediated via α receptors.

Anti-diuretic hormone (ADH or vasopressin) and angiotensin II are also powerful vasoconstrictor agents. In addition to its direct vasoconstrictor effects, angiotensin can also potentiate the effects of the sympathetic nerves. It does this by increasing the release of noradrenaline by adrenergic nerve terminals and by reducing the uptake of noradrenaline into them. A number of other substances can modulate the release or re-uptake of transmitters. Acetylcholine generally reduces the amount of noradrenaline released by nerve terminals. A similar inhibiting effect is exerted by ATP, ADP, adenosine, and, surprisingly, by noradrenaline, which, of course, has a direct vasoconstrictor action. Noradrenaline exerts its effect via α-receptors on the presynaptic endings of the nerve terminals. This negative feedback system may be important in limiting the output of noradrenaline at high frequencies of sympathetic discharge. Adrenaline acts via presynaptic β receptors to increase the output of transmitter from the nerve terminals. These potentiating effects of adrenaline via β receptors are seen at much lower concentrations than are the inhibitory effects of noradrenaline acting via α receptors on the presynaptic endings.

Further reading

Allen, J.M., Schon, F., Todd, N., Yeats, J.C., Crockard, H.A. & Bloom, S.R. (1984). Presence of Neuropeptide Y in human Circle of Willis and its possible role in cerebral vasospasm. *The Lancet*, September 1984.

Burnstock, G. (1980). Cholinergic and purinergic regulation of blood vessels. In: *Handbook of Physiology, Section 2, The Cardiovascular System*, Volume II, *Vascular Smooth Muscle*, pp. 567–612. American Physiological Society: Bethesda.

Keatinge, W.R. & Harman, M.C. (1980). *Local Mechanisms Controlling Blood Vessels*. Academic Press: London.

Rostere, W.H. (1984). Neurobiological and neuroendocrine functions of the vasoactive intestinal peptide (VIP). *Progress in Neurobiology*, 22, 103–29.

6

BLOOD FLOW TO DIFFERENT ORGANS AND TISSUES

In this chapter, I am going to discuss the structures and properties of the different circulations and how these differences relate to the functions of the different circulations. In considering different circulations, I shall discuss their properties from three viewpoints. Firstly, are there any special circumstances with which a particular circulation must cope? For example, the pulmonary circulation has to receive the whole of the cardiac output, which may vary between 5 and 25 litres every minute. Blood vessels within skeletal muscle and within the heart are going to be occluded when the muscle contracts. Hence, at the very time when the nutritive requirements of the muscle are greatest, that is, when the muscle is contracting most forcibly, the occlusion of the blood vessels will be greatest.

Secondly, I shall discuss the functions of the different circulations. One function of all systemic circulations is to supply oxygen and nutrients to the tissues and to remove waste products. In some circulations, for example, those to the heart and skeletal muscle, blood flow is very precisely matched to the oxygen needs of the tissue. However, this nutritive function is by no means the only function of many circulations. For example, the pulmonary circulation is concerned with the oxygenation of blood returning from the tissues, the bronchial arteries supplying nutrition to the airways and much of the connective tissue within the lungs. Blood flow to the skin is determined mainly by the thermoregulatory needs of the body and, in a warm environment, is greatly in excess of the metabolic needs of the skin. In the kidney at all times, and in the gastro-intestinal tract after a meal, blood flow vastly exceeds that needed for nutrition so that substances can be reabsorbed into the blood. Similarly, when glands are active, their blood flow becomes enormous so that the substances secreted can be carried in the blood.

Thirdly, I shall consider how the structure and arrangement of the blood vessels is related to the differing functions that the circulations have to perform and then discuss the different regulatory mechanisms by which blood flow is diverted from one region to another or within a tissue or organ.

6.1 The pulmonary circulation

The pulmonary circulation differs in many ways from other systemic circulations. The entire cardiac output is pumped through the pulmonary circulation. Mixed venous blood flows in the pulmonary artery to the lungs. Within the lungs, the blood is oxygenated and carbon dioxide is removed and the oxygenated blood returns to the left atrium via the pulmonary veins. The lungs receive a blood supply far in excess of their metabolic requirements. In fact, the metabolic needs of the airways and supporting tissues within the lungs are met by a supply of oxygenated blood from the bronchial arteries.

Pressures in the pulmonary arteries are very much lower than the average values of about 120 mmHg during systole and 80 mmHg during diastole found in large systemic arteries. Systolic pressures vary between 20 and 25 mmHg and diastolic pressures between 6 and 12 mmHg. Thus mean values for arterial pressure are between 10 and 15 mmHg.

Since the flows through the pulmonary and systemic circulations are the same, the low pressure in the pulmonary circulation must be associated with a much reduced resistance. The low resistance in the pulmonary circulation compared to the systemic circulation is due to structural differences in the vessels in the two regions. Pulmonary arteries and arterioles are shorter, thinner-walled and wider than their counterparts in the systemic circulation. The capillaries, too, are shorter and wider. Both arteries, arterioles and veins have less muscle in their walls than have systemic vessels. In the systemic circulation most of the resistance is provided by the arterioles which contain a great deal of smooth muscle in their walls. The much thinner-walled arterioles in the pulmonary circulation do not offer the same degree of resistance. In the pulmonary circulation the resistance seems to be distributed more evenly throughout the circulation with arteries, capillaries and veins all offering resistance to blood flow. Since resistance is fairly evenly distributed across the circulation the mean pressure in the capillaries (7–8 mmHg) is about half way between the pressure in the pulmonary artery (10–15 mmHg) and the pressure in the left atrium (2–5 mmHg).

These structural features of pulmonary vessels mean that the compliance (that is, the change in volume for a given change in pressure) of the pulmonary circulation is high (3 ml per mmHg change in pressure) — a value which almost equals that of the systemic circulation as a whole. Thus, pulmonary vessels are highly distensible and have an important capacitance function. Capacitance in the pulmonary circulation is provided approximately equally by the arterial and the venous sides of the circulation rather than mainly by the veins as it is in the systemic circulation.

This low pressure in the pulmonary circulation has a number of important effects. Firstly, it means that the right ventricle is pumping against a lower pressure and therefore does less work than the left ventricle. Secondly, it means that mean capillary hydrostatic pressure (7–8 mmHg) is less than the plasma oncotic pressure. In the lungs, the hydrostatic pressure outside the capillaries is normally equal to alveolar pressure which is normally close to atmospheric pressure. Thus, the hydrostatic pressure difference acting to force fluid out is normally less than the oncotic forces drawing fluid in so fluid is reabsorbed along the whole length of the capillary rather than being filtered at the arterial end and reabsorbed at the venous end of the capillary as occurs in systemic capillaries (see Section 4.2.3). The oncotic forces pulling fluid into the blood vessels are so strong that the pulmonary interstitial space is reduced to almost nothing. This is physiologically significant as it reduces the distance over which oxygen has to diffuse. It is also an important mechanism for keeping the alveoli dry. A rise in pulmonary arterial pressure to a level which exceeds oncotic pressure and the subsequent accumulation of fluid in the interstitial spaces will therefore make diffusion more difficult and may result in the accumulation of fluid within the alveoli. There is, however, a large safety factor before pulmonary oedema will occur as a result of a rise in pulmonary arterial pressure. The capillary pressure has to rise from a resting value of about 8 mmHg to exceed the oncotic pressure of 25 mmHg before pulmonary oedema will occur. During chronic elevation of pulmonary arterial pressure, flow in the lymphatics increases, removing some of the fluid from the interstitial spaces.

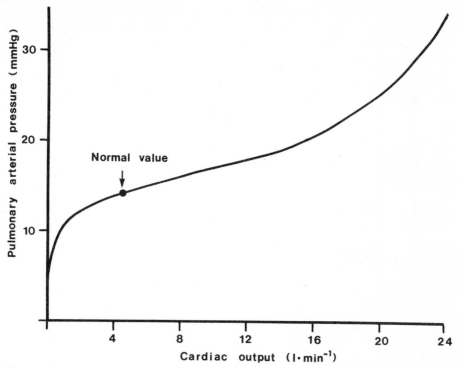

Figure 6.1. The effect of raising cardiac output on pulmonary arterial pressure.

The high distensibility of the vessels within the pulmonary circulation means that the lungs can act as a reservoir for blood. When cardiac output increases blood can be 'milked' from the pulmonary circulation to maintain filling of the left side of the heart for a few beats until the systemic venous return increases to match the increased output from the heart. Large shifts in blood flow from the pulmonary to the systemic circulations can occur when a subject expires hard against a resistance, for example, when blowing a trumpet or performing the Valsalva manoeuvre (see Section 10.3).

Large changes in blood flow to the lungs cause minimal changes in the pulmonary arterial pressure (see Figure 6.1). This is because as flow increases the resistance to blood flow in the pulmonary circulation falls. At low arterial pressures this is due to the opening up of vessels within the circulation which are normally closed. At higher arterial pressures, the fall in resistance is due to distension of the vessels. At very high values of cardiac output, pulmonary arterial pressure rises steeply (see Figure 6.1). If pulmonary arterial pressure rises to a level which exceeds the oncotic pressure then pulmonary oedema will occur.

Some increase in the pressure within the left atrium may also occur without a resultant increase in pulmonary arterial pressure (see Figure 6.2). Again this is due to the opening up of vessels within the lungs which are normally closed. An increase in left atrial pressure outside the normal range, as occurs in left heart failure, will result in a rise in pulmonary arterial pressure and possibly lead to pulmonary oedema.

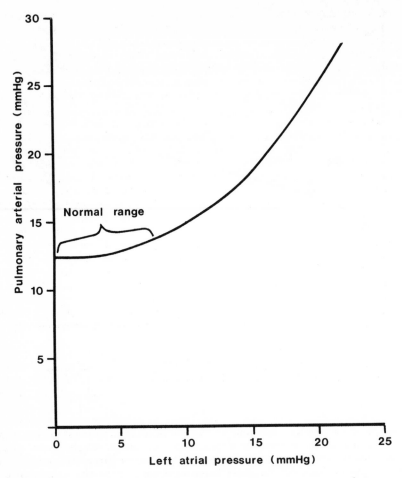

Figure 6.2. The effect of raising left atrial pressure on pulmonary arterial pressure.

There is an uneven distribution of blood flow within the lungs. In the upright position, mean pulmonary arterial pressure at the apices of the lungs is about 3 mmHg, at the level of the heart is about 13 mmHg and at the base of the lungs is about 21 mmHg. As a result of these differences in pressure, blood flow at the base of the lungs is about ten times greater than that at the apex. In fact, the perfusing pressure at the apices of the lungs is so low that blood flows only during systole. During situations such as heavy exercise, when pulmonary vascular pressure rises, the capillaries at the apices of the lungs will be open and blood will flow to all regions of the lung, although the blood flow to the base will still exceed that to the apices. In the supine position, the pressure gradients between the apices and the base of the lungs are removed but here the posterior aspects of the lungs receive a greater blood flow than the anterior regions. In the upright posture, ventilation at the base of the lungs is about twice that at the apices, but there remains a mismatch between ventilation and perfusion.

Local mechanisms in the lungs operate to try to minimise inequalities of ventilation and perfusion. If ventilation is reduced relative to perfusion, then the alveolar partial pressure of oxygen (PO_2) will fall and the alveolar partial pressure of carbon dioxide (PCO_2) will rise. This will produce both a relaxation of the smooth muscle within the bronchioles (reducing airway resistance and increasing ventilation) and a vasoconstriction of the smooth muscle in the arterioles (reducing blood flow to the region). Bronchial smooth muscle seems to be influenced more by the partial pressure of carbon dioxide than of oxygen and the smooth muscle in the blood vessels is influenced more by hypoxia. This vasoconstriction of blood vessels in response to hypoxia is the opposite of the effect seen in the systemic circulation (see Section 5.2). The difference between the effects of hypoxia on arterioles in the systemic and pulmonary circulations is of functional significance. In the systemic circulation, hypoxia results in an increase in the blood flow to the tissues and hence an increase in the supply of oxygen to that tissue. In the pulmonary circulation, however, hypoxia results in a reduction in the blood flow to that region of the lung and thus limits the perfusion of areas of the lung which are inadequately ventilated. It is the PO_2 in the alveoli rather than in the blood which is important. It is not yet known whether hypoxia exerts its effects on blood vessels by a direct action or via the release of a vasoactive substance or substances. A number of substances which are vasodilators in the systemic circulation produce a vasoconstriction in the pulmonary circulation. These substances include the kinins and histamine although, as yet, there is no firm evidence to support a role for any of these substances in mediating the vasoconstriction induced by hypoxia.

The arterioles and arteries within the pulmonary circulation are supplied with sympathetic vasoconstrictor fibres. However, these nerves have a very much smaller effect on the resistance to blood flow in the pulmonary circulation than, for example, in the circulation to the skeletal muscle. Maximal stimulation of these nerves results in only about a 30 per cent increase in resistance. This may be, at least in part, because some of the resistance to flow in the pulmonary circulation lies in the capillaries which do not receive an innervation from sympathetic vasoconstrictor fibres. Although the sympathetic nerves have little effect on resistance in the pulmonary circulation, they do have important effects on the capacitance of the circulation. The major control of pulmonary blood flow is an intrinsic regulatory system based on oxygen. Oxygen regulates its own uptake by adjusting local perfusion to match local ventilation.

6.2 The coronary circulation

The heart has a high blood flow at rest (approximately 60–80 ml·min^{-1}·100g^{-1}.) Although there is a dense capillary network, there may be few collaterals or linking vessels between the large vessels so in the event of a vessel becoming obstructed, the area supplied by that vessel will become ischaemic. In the smaller vessels, collaterals may open up several hours after occlusion of a vessel. Thus, not only must the total coronary blood flow be maintained as a high priority, but the blood must also be distributed throughout the coronary network.

The major problem that the coronary circulation has to overcome is that coronary vessels, particularly those supplying the left ventricle, are occluded during systole (see Figure 6.3). About 80 per cent of the blood flow to the muscle of the left ventricle occurs during diastole. When the heart is

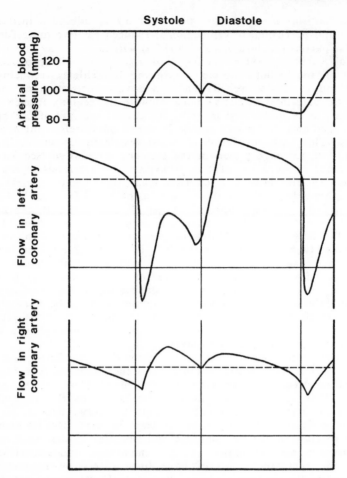

Figure 6.3. Changes in arterial blood pressure and blood flow in the left and right coronary arteries during a cardiac cycle. The unbroken horizontal lines represent the point at which no flow occurs and the dotted lines represent the mean values for pressure and flow.

contracting strongly there may be a complete cessation of flow in the left coronary artery during systole. In a healthy subject, with a normal resting heart rate, this reduction in flow during systole is not a problem since the period of diastole is long enough to provide an adequate blood flow. Problems may arise, however, when heart rate increases. This increases the oxygen demand of the heart but, by reducing the diastolic period, reduces the time available for blood flow to the heart muscle to take place.

Blood flow to the heart is very closely linked to the oxygen requirement of the heart (see Figure 6.4) and, in very heavy exercise, may increase to as much as 300 ml·min^{-1}·100g^{-1}. Hypoxia and, to a lesser extent, local metabolites (including carbon dioxide and hydrogen ions) are important in producing vasodilatation of the resistance vessels. It has not been established whether the lack of oxygen acts directly on the walls of the blood vessels or whether

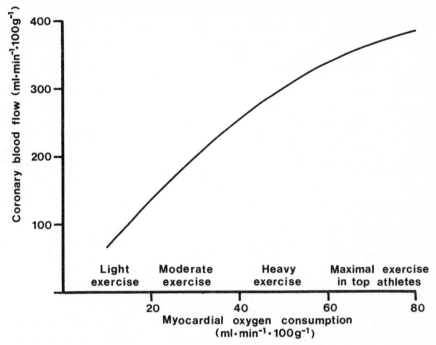

Figure 6.4. The relationship between coronary blood flow and the oxygen consumption of the heart.

the vasodilatation is brought about by an intermediary. The latter seems more likely and adenosine has been suggested as the intermediary. Coronary blood flow will increase when the oxygen consumption of the heart increases. Increases in heart rate will result in a greater demand for oxygen (and hence for blood) than will increases in stroke volume produced by inotropic effects on the heart (see Section 3.3).

Stimulation of the sympathetic nerves to the heart results in an increase in coronary blood flow. Therefore it was suggested that, in the coronary vessels, sympathetic nerves have a direct vasodilator action. However, stimulation of the sympathetic nerves to the heart also increases heart rate and the force of contraction of the heart. This leads to an increase in the oxygen consumption of the heart and, consequently, an increase in coronary blood flow. When these effects on the rate and force of contraction of the heart are eliminated by giving β-adrenoreceptor blocking drugs, sympathetic stimulation results in vasoconstriction, as it does in most circulations. However, under normal circumstances this small, direct vasoconstrictor effect is masked by the larger, indirect vasodilatation resulting from the heart's increased oxygen consumption.

There is evidence of some tonic sympathetic vasoconstrictor discharge to blood vessels in the coronary circulation. However, the significance of the direct effects of the sympathetic nerves on coronary blood vessels remains obscure. It has been suggested that the attacks of anginal pain (caused by an inadequate coronary blood flow) which are experienced by some patients with coronary artery disease on exposure to a cold wind may be due to a reflex-induced sympathetic vasoconstriction of the coronary blood vessels in response to the cold. The direct and indirect effects of adrenaline both result in a vasodilatation, the direct effects being mediated via β-adrenoreceptors.

Coronary arteries also receive a parasympathetic nerve supply but its functional significance remains unclear. Reflex cholinergic vasodilatation of the coronary vessels may be important in pathological conditions such as myocardial infarction, when the cardiac C fibres (see Section 7.2.2) can be activated.

Coronary artery disease is a major cause of death in western society. Therefore, it is important that the physiological principles underlying the treatment of patients with coronary insufficiency are understood. The oxygen supply to the heart can be related by the Fick principle to the amount of oxygen extracted by the heart and the coronary blood flow. In cardiac muscle, the extraction of oxygen is normally high. There is some evidence that the oxygen extraction of patients with ischaemic hearts can be increased by an exercise regime but the rationale behind most of the treatments for coronary artery disease is either to increase the blood flow or, more often, to lower the oxygen demand of the heart.

Blood flow to the heart will depend upon the pressure gradient across the circulation and the resistance to blood flow. The pressure gradient could potentially be increased by increasing aortic pressure but, since this will also increase the oxygen demand of the heart, it is not a useful approach. Resistance to blood flow, according to the Hagen—Poiseuille equation is mainly determined by the radius of the vessels. Thus, one way of increasing blood flow is to widen the vessels. This can potentially be done by using drugs which remove deposits occluding the inside of the vessels, using drugs which dilate the coronary vessels or by replacing occluded vessels with vessels which have a larger internal diameter.

An alternative approach is to accept that coronary blood flow is reduced and alter the oxygen demand of the heart instead. Vasodilator drugs mainly work in this way, since by reducing aortic pressure they reduce the work of the heart. This indirect effect is probably more important than any possible direct effects of these drugs on the coronary vessels. Sympathetic blocking drugs, such as the β-adrenoreceptor blocking drugs, by reducing the heart rate and force of contraction of the heart and, ultimately, the aortic pressure, will reduce the oxygen consumption of the heart at rest. More importantly, they will limit the increase in oxygen demand that can occur, for example, during exercise or emotion. The reduction in heart rate produced by these drugs is particularly important because it increases the period during which blood can flow to the heart.

Patients with coronary artery disease will seek advice from their doctors on what activities they should avoid. From our knowledge of the factors influencing the oxygen consumption of the heart (see Section 3.3), it is clear that increases in heart rate and blood pressure are potentially the most dangerous. Thus, it is often advisable for patients to undertake a mild form of exercise rather than to watch, with excitement or frustration, their favourite football team play.

The heart has its own protective mechanisms which come into play when areas of the muscle become ischaemic. The free nerve endings giving rise to C fibres (see Section 7.2.2) are stimulated and result in hypotension and bradycardia mediated by an increased vagal activity to the heart. These changes reduce the work of the heart and, hence, the demand for oxygen and blood.

6.3 The cerebral circulation

The cerebral circulation shares many of the properties of the coronary circulation. Both have a high blood flow at rest which must be maintained, so both are high-priority circulations. In both circulations, there are important protective reflexes which help to maintain the blood flow if the tissue becomes ischaemic.

There are a number of structural peculiarities in the cerebral circulation. Firstly, because the brain is surrounded by a rigid cranium in the adult, the combined volume of the brain tissue, cerebrospinal fluid and intracranial blood is nearly constant. Total cerebral blood flow remains fairly constant at about 50–60 $ml\cdot min^{-1}\cdot 100g^{-1}$. Secondly, the walls of the capillaries are specialised to act as a barrier to prevent some substances entering the brain. In general, lipid-soluble molecules, such as carbon dioxide, readily enter the brain. Some substances, such as glucose and amino acids, have special carrier mechanisms to allow them to enter the brain. Other substances, for example, many elemental ions, cross the blood–brain barrier only with difficulty. The blood supply to the brain is via the vertebral and internal carotid arteries and, although there are connections between these vessels at the circle of Willis, occlusion of one of these vessels results in ischaemia of that part of the brain which it supplies.

Total blood flow to the brain is relatively constant and there is evidence of pronounced autoregulation in response to changes in perfusion pressure. There are, however, important differences in the distribution of blood flow within the brain. When one area of the brain is metabolically active, blood flow to

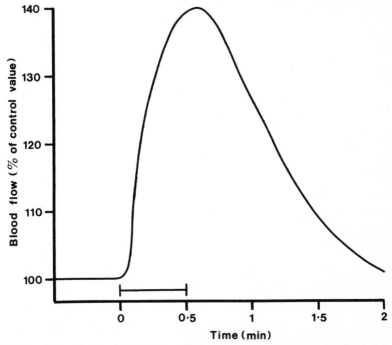

Figure 6.5. The effect of shining a light on the retina (as indicated by the horizontal bar) on the blood flow to the visual cortex.

that region increases. For example, blood flow to the visual cortex increases when a light is shone on the retina (see Figure 6.5). It is generally accepted that these changes in blood flow are mediated by the release of vasodilator metabolites. Adenosine and potassium ions are possible candidates but hypoxia and increases in PCO_2 or hydrogen ion concentration ($[H^+]$) may also be important. The concentration of hydrogen ions in the brain can also alter with ventilation. During hyperventilation, carbon dioxide is blown off so arterial PCO_2 falls. Since CO_2 crosses the blood brain barrier readily, is hydrated and dissociates into H^+ and HCO_3-, $[H^+]$ in the interstitium will fall and the resultant vasoconstriction will result in ischaemia of the brain tissue and a sensation of dizziness. In addition, cerebral blood vessels dilate in response to hypoxia so ventilation with gas mixtures rich in oxygen will cause cerebral vasoconstriction.

Blood vessels within the brain are innervated by sympathetic vasoconstrictor nerve fibres which have very little tonic activity. They may also be innervated by cholinergic and peptidergic fibres, although the role of these two types of fibres is obscure. In cerebral vessels, the receptors are less sensitive to noradrenaline than are receptors in other vessels, for example, in the blood vessels supplying skeletal muscle. Under normal conditions, stimulation of the sympathetic nerves has little or no effect on cerebral blood flow. However, in the face of a sudden increase in arterial pressure, sympathetic vasoconstriction may be seen, and will have a protective function. Thus, normally, blood flow within the brain is controlled by local metabolic factors.

As in the heart, important protective mechanisms exist to safeguard the blood supply to the brain in the event of brain tissue becoming ischaemic. If intracranial pressure rises, for example, because of the growth of a tumour in the brain, then this increase in pressure will tend to occlude the blood vessels. As a result of the tissue ischaemia, changes in the activity of neurones within the brain will produce a very powerful activation of the sympathetic preganglionic neurones which supply blood vessels in all regions, including the kidney. The subsequent powerful peripheral vasoconstriction will result in an increase in the systemic blood pressure and, thus, an increase in the pressure within the cerebral vessels. If the pressure within the vessels exceeds the intracranial pressure then the cerebral blood vessels will re-open and normal blood flow will be restored. This large increase in blood pressure and the associated reflex bradycardia mediated by the baroreceptors (see Section 7.1) are important clinical signs of a potentially dangerous increase in intracranial pressure.

6.4 The skeletal muscle circulation

In skeletal muscle also, blood flow varies depending upon the metabolic needs of the tissue. There are two types of skeletal muscle: tonic and phasic. Tonic muscles make up about 10–20 per cent of the muscle mass in man and are concerned with the maintenance of posture. They are continuously active and cannot sustain an oxygen debt. The oxygen requirements of these tonic muscles are higher than those of the phasic muscles. The muscle is more vascular and has a resting blood flow which is about three times greater and also varies less than that of phasic muscles.

The bulk of the muscle mass is phasic muscle which has a low blood flow at rest (about 2–5 ml·min^{-1}·100g^{-1}). When phasic muscle contracts blood flow to the muscle is increased, but during the contractions blood flow is occluded as it is in the heart during systole. However, this is less of a problem than it is in the heart because phasic muscle is able to sustain an oxygen debt between contractions.

The relationship between oxygen consumption and blood flow in skeletal muscle during muscular exercise is similar to that in the heart. Blood flow in denervated limbs increases during exercise so it is thought that local factors are important in regulating blood flow. There has been a number of attempts to isolate the 'key metabolite' responsible for the pronounced vasodilatation which occurs during exercise. Many substances have been cited as potentially fulfilling this role, of which potassium ions and an increase in the osmolality of the blood have attracted most attention. However, in order to fulfil this role, the putative key metabolite must be shown to be able to mimic the vasodilatation of exercise at the concentration at which it is found during exercise. The concentration of extracellular potassium ions ($[K^+]$) rises at the start of exercise to levels which would produce a considerable vasodilatation and thus it is thought to be important in mediating the vasodilatation which occurs in the first few minutes of exercise. Increases in osmotic pressure, caused by the breakdown of glycogen to smaller molecules, may also be of importance in moderate or heavy exercise. However, in mild exercise osmotic pressure does not increase appreciably so some other factor must be responsible for the vasodilatation seen in mild exercise. Neither an increase in $[K^+]$ nor an increase in osmotic pressure play an important role in the vasodilatation occurring in the latter stages of exercise.

To summarise, the vasodilatation in skeletal muscle can be largely, but not completely, explained in terms of changes in $[K^+]$, osmotic pressure, hypoxia, PCO_2 and $[H^+]$ but there are probably additional factors of importance which are yet to be identified. Certainly, there is no single substance which can explain the vasodilatation which occurs in all the different stages and intensities of exercise.

Nerves and hormones can also alter the radius of blood vessels in skeletal muscle. There is a sympathetic vasoconstrictor supply to the blood vessels which is tonically active. This tonic discharge is greater in the erect posture because of the effects mediated by the baroreceptors (see Section 9.1). Sectioning these nerves results in an increase in blood flow to a new resting value of between 6 and 9 ml·min^{-1}·100g^{-1}. Thus, a withdrawal of some of this discharge would result in vasodilatation. Stimulation of sympathetic cholinergic nerves results in vasodilatation of the blood vessels during the defence reaction but their possible involvement in the vasodilatation which occurs during exercise remains a subject for speculation. These nervous influences are likely to be of importance only in the early stages or in anticipation of exercise. Adrenaline, released from the adrenal medulla and acting via β receptors, will also contribute to the vasodilatation which occurs during exercise in skeletal muscle.

Thus, blood flow to the heart, brain and skeletal muscle is very closely linked to the nutritive requirements of the tissues and is controlled largely by local factors. I will now discuss a group of systemic circulations whose flow is governed mainly by influences other than the nutritive needs of the tissues.

6.5 The cutaneous circulation

The skin has a particular problem as it is the part of the body which is subjected to the greatest extremes of temperature and various types of trauma.

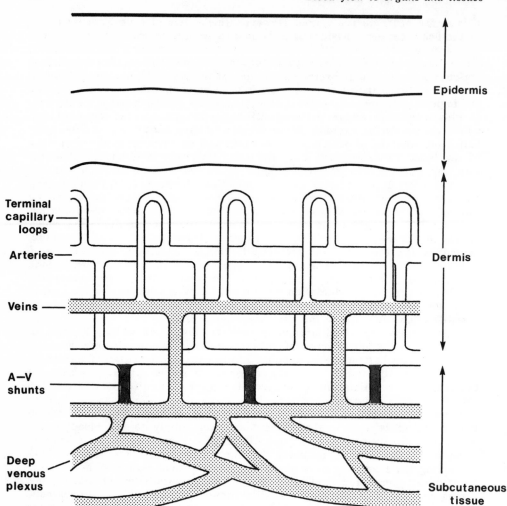

Figure 6.6. The arrangement of blood vessels within the skin.

The major function of the circulation to the skin is a thermoregulatory one. Blood flow is increased so that heat can be lost from the body and decreased so that heat loss from the skin can be minimised and body heat maintained.

There are structural peculiarities in the blood vessels in the skin which are related to the skin's thermoregulatory function. In areas of the skin where the ratio of surface area to volume is large, such as the fingers, toes, ears and face, thick-walled vessels — the arteriovenous (A–V) anastomoses or shunts — are present (see Figure 6.6). These vessels directly link the arterioles and venules, by-passing the capillary network. They have a dense supply of sympathetic vasoconstrictor nerve fibres and small changes in the discharge of these nerves have a very profound effect on the blood flow through the A–V anastomoses.

The most efficient heat exchange occurs in the terminal capillary loops that lie close to the skin surface. Here, the temperature gradient from blood to tissue is greatest because the tissue temperature is close to that of the environment and the high surface area to volume ratio favours heat exchange. However, there is a limit to the amount of heat which can be lost via the capillaries. The A—V anastomoses provide a further mechanism for losing heat from the body. When the A—V anastomoses open, the deep venous plexi in the dermis are filled with warm blood and heat can be lost from these vessels to the environment.

In the limbs, the arteries supplying the extremities have accompanying veins which act as counter-current heat exchangers. In cold environmental temperatures, the cold blood returning from the extremities helps to lower the temperature of the arterial blood travelling to the extremities, minimising heat loss from the body. This arrangement of vessels also means that blood returning to the heart is warmed.

Blood flow in the skin is largely determined by the thermoregulatory needs of the body. Naked man is in thermoequilibrium when the environmental temperature is between 25 and 30°C. At this temperature, average skin blood flow is about 20 $ml·min^{-1}·100g^{-1}$ and there is still some tonic sympathetic vasoconstrictor discharge to the vessels. When the vessels are denervated, blood flow to parts of the skin which have few A—V shunts only rises to about 25—30 $ml·min^{-1}·100g^{-1}$ but in areas where there is a considerable number of A—V shunts, blood flow may rise to as high as 60—80 $ml·min^{-1}·100g^{-1}$. This is because the walls of the A—V shunts contain no elastic tissue. The smooth muscle in their walls has little myogenic activity and is dominated by the sympathetic vasoconstrictor nerves rather than by local factors. In areas of the skin where A—V shunts are not present, the arterioles do possess myogenic activity and their radius is not so dominated by activity of the sympathetic vasoconstrictor fibres. This myogenic activity can be demonstrated by firmly stroking the skin of the back of the hand with a blunt instrument. A localised vasoconstriction, the white reaction, can be seen after a few seconds which lasts for about a minute.

Changes in the level of discharge of the sympathetic vasoconstrictor fibres are brought about by the heat gain and heat loss centres in the hypothalamus. In response to a rise in the environmental temperature, there is first a withdrawal of the tonic vasoconstrictor discharge to the A—V shunts in the ears and hands and then in the feet. This is followed by a more general vasodilatation and venodilatation. If the heat stress is sufficient to induce sweating, then there will be an increase in the blood flow to sweat glands in order to supply the raw materials for the production of sweat. In extreme heat stress, blood flow to the skin may reach levels of as high as 150 $ml·min^{-1}·100g^{-1}$. In this case, vasodilatation is mediated by the release of bradykinin or a similar local hormone and is secondary to the activation of the sweat glands. A similar mechanism may be responsible for the increase in blood flow which occurs during emotional sweating.

Increases in sympathetic vasoconstrictor discharge will occur when the environmental temperature falls and can reduce the average skin blood flow to less than 1 $ml·min^{-1}·100g^{-1}$. Changes in skin blood flow are also seen as a result of local changes in the skin temperature. The initial response to immersion of one hand in cold water is a marked vasoconstriction which can be maintained for up to ten minutes. On prolonged immersion in cold water, cold vasodilatation occurs (see Section 5.2). A smaller and solely reflex vasoconstriction of the blood vessels in the warm hand is also seen (see Figure 6.7).

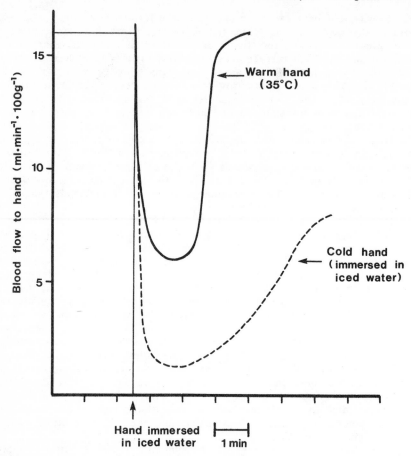

Figure 6.7. The effect of immersion of one hand in iced water on the blood flow to both hands.

As long as the skin temperature does not drop sufficiently low as to induce cold vasodilatation, the sympathetic vasoconstrictor activity to skin vessels is maintained. Thus, the phenomenon of 'autoregulatory escape' as occurs in the intestine (see Section 6.7), in which the build-up of metabolites produces a vasodilatation which overrides the reflex-induced vasoconstriction, is not seen. This is partly because, on exposure to the cold, the metabolic requirements of the skin also fall.

Reductions in skin blood flow may also occur in other circumstances, for example, in response to blood loss. These changes are brought about by an increase in the discharge of the sympathetic vasoconstrictor fibres innervating the blood vessels. The release of adrenaline, which in the skin only acts on α-adrenergic receptors on the blood vessels, will also contribute to this vasoconstriction after haemorrhage.

Marked changes in skin blood flow also occur in response to cutaneous trauma or allergic reactions. The triple response which occurs when the skin is subjected to trauma was described by Lewis in 1927. The components of this triple response are:

(1) The red reaction — a local vasodilatation of the precapillary vessels due to the release of histamine or other local hormones

(2) The wheal — local oedema resulting from the increase in capillary permeability caused by the release of local hormones

(3) The flare — a more widespread vasodilatation of the precapillary vessels, possibly mediated by local axon reflexes and involving nociceptive fibres (see Section 5.3).

External pressure on the skin producing ischaemia of the tissues will result in an increase in the blood flow to the skin when the pressure is removed. However, a prolonged interruption of flow to an area of skin will cause tissue damage, for example, bed sores. During normal sleep, changes in body position occur and prevent the prolonged interruption of blood flow to particular areas of skin.

6.6 The renal circulation

The two main functions of the kidney are to remove unwanted materials from the body (excretion) and to regulate the composition and volume of the body fluids (homeostatis). In order that the kidney can carry out these functions, it receives a blood flow which is far in excess of its metabolic needs, approximately 400 ml·min^{-1}·100g^{-1}.

Both the structure and arrangement of blood vessels within the kidney are of considerable functional significance. Within the kidney, the renal arteries branch successively and form the afferent arterioles which give rise to the glomerular capillaries. These capillaries then form a second set of arterioles, the efferent arterioles, whose capillaries (the peritubular capillaries) supply the different parts of the kidney tubules. Blood from these capillaries drains into the venous side of the renal circulation (see Figure 6.8). Thus, the kidney is an example of an organ having a portal system (see Section 1.2 for other examples). Pressure needs to be high at the glomerulus where filtration of plasma occurs but lower at the capillaries supplying the tubules where reabsorption and secretion can occur, allowing the fine control of the urinary excretion of different substances.

Blood enters the glomerular capillaries from the afferent arterioles and that which is not filtered out leaves the glomeruli via the efferent arterioles. The filtered fluid passes through the capillary endothelium, the basement membrane and the epithelium of Bowman's capsule before it enters the tubule. The glomerular capillaries are fenestrated, having large pores within their endothelium (see Section 4.2.3). This endothelial layer provides a barrier for the blood cells. The barrier to protein molecules is much more difficult to define; while on the basis of the size of the filtration pores, it was postulated that the basement membrane constitutes the major barrier, there is evidence that the negatively charged glycosidoproteins which coat the endothelium, the basement membrane and the epithelial cells of the Bowman's capsule contribute significantly to the barrier function. The area available for filtration at the glomerular capillaries is greater than that in many other capillaries.

The peritubular capillaries are like those in most other tissues. The reabsorption of fluid into these capillaries is not aided by any particular structural differences in the vessels but more by the large total surface area which they offer, the low capillary hydrostatic pressure and the higher-than-normal oncotic pressure of the plasma.

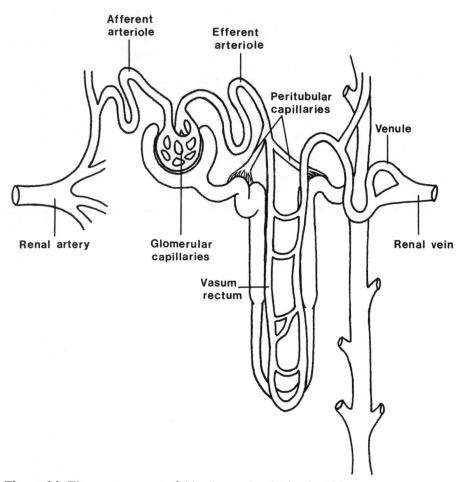

Figure 6.8. The arrangement of blood vessels within the kidney.

The structural arrangement of the vessels and their relationship to the kidney tubule also aids in the production of a concentrated urine. In the renal medulla, a high osmolality is created by the loops of Henle which act as counter-current multipliers. The loops of Henle dip down into the medulla and an area of high osmolality is created at their tips. If the blood vessels were to pass by the tips of these loops, then much of this increased osmolality would be lost into the blood. Instead, the blood vessels supplying the loops of Henle, the vasa recta, are arranged so that they too dip down into the medulla, following the loops of Henle. These vasa recta act as counter-current exchangers. Thus, the high osmolality created by the loops of Henle is retained in the medulla. When highly concentrated urine is being produced, anti-diuretic hormone is released which reduces blood flow within the vasa recta, aiding the production of concentrated urine.

Total renal blood flow remains relatively constant even in the face of changes in pressure over a wide range (80—160 mmHg). The precise mechanism whereby the kidney is able to autoregulate over this wide range of pressures is not clear. It is thought that, in addition to the increase in myogenic activity and the subsequent vasoconstriction of the afferent arteriole produced by stretching the vessel when blood pressure increases (see Section 5.2), there may be other mechanisms. There may be a feedback between the distal part of the tubule and the afferent arteriole, known as the tubulo-glomerular feedback. An increase in the amount of fluid delivered to the distal tubule may be monitored by cells of the macula densa and could result in a vasoconstriction of the afferent arteriole. The effector mechanisms remain unclear although one possibility is that the renin-angiotensin system acts as the link. A possible role for adenosine has also been suggested although the evidence for such a mechanism is scanty.

Although total renal blood flow does remain relatively constant, it may be influenced by changes in the discharge of the sympathetic efferent nerves to the blood vessels. A small decrease in sympathetic discharge induced, for example, by stimulation of atrial receptors or C fibres within the heart (see Section 7.2) may result in a small increase in the renal blood flow. More striking changes are seen during the defence reaction (see Section 8.1) and cerebral ischaemia (see Section 6.3). In both these situations, there is a very powerful sympathetic vasoconstriction which is particularly pronounced during cerebral ischaemia when the maintenance of blood flow to the kidney is no longer a high priority. There is also some evidence of an innervation of renal blood vessels by cholinergic nerves and by dopaminergic nerves although their function has yet to be elucidated.

Many substances, including hormones, local hormones and peptides can also affect renal blood flow but the functional significance of these mechanisms remains unclear. It may be that one of the hormones released by the gastro-intestinal tract is responsible for the increase in blood flow in the kidney which follows a meal.

Since the kidney's total blood flow is vastly in excess of its nutritive needs, blood flow is not influenced by changes in metabolism in the kidney, that is, local metabolic factors are unimportant in determining total blood flow.

Although total blood flow remains relatively constant, there are important changes in the distribution of blood flow to different parts of the kidney. These can be brought about by both nerves and hormones. Blood flow to the outer cortical areas of the kidney normally vastly exceeds that to the inner medulla. Shifts can occur in the distribution of blood flow between cortex and medulla. Sympathetic nerves innervate both the afferent and efferent arterioles and can, therefore, affect both filtration and reabsorption by altering blood flow through these two sets of vessels. Sympathetic discharge also releases renin from the juxtaglomerular apparatus. This may result in a redistribution of renal blood flow since angiotensin affects the efferent arterioles more than the afferent arterioles. Evidence of the precise effects of local hormones, for example, prostaglandins and kinins, on intra-renal blood flow distribution remains scanty, but these substances may well have physiologically significant effects.

6.7 The splanchnic circulation

The circulation to the gastro-intestinal tract, including the liver and pancreas, is often referred to as the splanchnic circulation. Blood flow in the splanchnic circulation, as in the kidney, is not determined by the metabolic needs of the tissue. The blood flow requirements of the gastro-intestinal tract will vary depending on the motility of the gut, the rate of secretion from the glands and the rate of absorption from the gut mucosa.

At rest, blood flow to the gut is approximately $15–40$ ml·min^{-1}·100g^{-1}, although there is some regional variation. For example, resting blood flow to the salivary glands is about $20–25$ ml·min^{-1}·100g^{-1}, to the stomach and small intestine about $20–40$ ml·min^{-1}·100g^{-1} and to the large intestine $15–25$ ml·min^{-1}·100g^{-1}. These figures are very approximate and a large range of values has been described in different studies. The blood vessels supplying the mucosa, submucosa and muscle seem to be arranged in parallel with a far greater blood flow going to the mucosa than to the smooth muscle.

The gastro-intestinal tract is linked to the liver via the portal vein. There have also been suggestions that other portal systems exist within the gastro-intestinal tract. A portal system linking the duodenum and pancreas, with a function similar to that of the hypophyseal portal system (that is, the transport of hormones from their site of release to their site of action without them entering the general circulation) has been suggested but there is little evidence for this. Portal systems within the salivary glands have also been suggested, but their existence is not universally accepted. There is evidence of a portal system within the pancreas itself linking the islets of Langerhans and the exocrine tissue of the gland. It has been suggested that the insulin, glucagon and somatostatin, released by the islet cells and present in high concentrations in the portal blood, modulate secretion from the exocrine part of the pancreas.

There is a great deal of controversy over the existence of a counter-current exchange system associated with the villi of the mucosa of the small intestine, which would have a similar function to the vasa recta associated with the loops of Henle in the kidney (see Section 6.6). The anatomical arrangement of the blood vessels supplying the villi is such that counter-current exchange could exist. In fact, if blood is to reach the tip of the villi and return to the heart such an anatomical arrangement must occur. On first examination, the role of a counter-current exchanger system seems questionable. The formation of a region of high osmolality at the tip of a villus may hinder intestinal absorption. Advocates of the counter-current exchange theory have suggested that the system works either to aid water absorption, as it does in the kidney, or to limit the rate at which absorbed substances enter the blood. Such a system would, of course, mean that oxygen in the arterial blood would by-pass the tip of the villi. It has been suggested that the rapid turnover of epithelial cells at the tips of the villi provides evidence in support of a poor delivery of oxygen to the tips of the villi resulting from the existence of a counter-current mechanism. At a high blood flow, for example, following a meal, little exchange would occur across the vessels. It is difficult to see the function of a counter-current exchange system which operates primarily in the fasting state.

The intestinal vascular bed shows pronounced autoregulation in the face of changes in perfusion pressure. This is particularly important in organs such as the intestine, pancreas and salivary glands which have fenestrated capillary beds, since, in the capillaries, the maintenance of a steady level of capillary pressure is essential in order to prevent oedema (Section 4.2.3).

Following a meal, total blood flow to the gastro-intestinal tract doubles or trebles, but it does so in a sequential manner and the increase is particularly marked in the stomach and small intestine. The mechanisms responsible for this increase in blood flow remain unclear and probably differ from one part of the gastro-intestinal tract to another. In the salivary glands, during secretion, blood flow increases enormously (approximately thirty fold), reaching values as high as 700 ml·min^{-1}·100g^{-1}. Stimulation of the vagal nerves increases secretion and blood flow. There has been much discussion as to whether the vagal nerves have a direct effect on the blood vessels or act via some intermediary. In the case of the salivary glands, an important role was once thought to be played by the powerful vasodilator peptide, kallidin, which is formed from its precursor kininogen by the action of kallikrein released during secretion. However, other regulatory peptides, for example, VIP, are now thought to be important. The discovery of these mechanisms does not deny the existence of a direct vasodilator action of the vagal nerves on the blood vessels.

Similarly, in the stomach, whenever secretion is stimulated there is an associated increase in blood flow up to about 150 $ml·min^{-1}·100g^{-1}$. This may be mediated either via the release of peptides produced by the action of the vagal nerves on the myenteric plexus or via a common intermediary which is responsible for both the increase in secretion and the increase in blood flow. In the small intestine, the increase in blood flow seen after a meal is unlikely to be mediated by a direct effect of the vagal nerves on the blood vessels. In the small intestine, blood flow to both the mucosa and the muscle increases greatly but, as in the stomach, the increase in blood flow is greater to the glands than to the smooth muscle. Blood flow to the large intestine varies very much less after a meal and there is again no evidence for a direct effect of the vagal nerves on the blood vessels. In the pancreas, also, there does not seem to be a direct innervation of the blood vessels by the vagal nerves. Thus, the small increase in blood flow which occurs on vagal stimulation of the pancreas may be mediated by the actions of kinins or result from the increased metabolism of the secretory cells. Secretin may also enhance blood flow slightly. Changes in pancreatic blood flow are very much less than those seen in, for example, the stomach.

In summary, blood flow to the gut increases following a meal but it is not yet clear whether this hyperaemia is mediated by a direct effect of the parasympathetic vasodilator nerves or by hormones or regulatory peptides which are also released following a meal. The mechanisms may well differ from one part of the gut to another.

Changes in gut motility would be expected to influence the blood flow to the smooth muscle but the difficulties of investigating motility without associated changes in secretion mean that little research has been done on this subject.

Stimulation of the sympathetic nerves to blood vessels within the gastro-intestinal tract results in an initial pronounced vasoconstriction but this is not maintained. After about a minute blood flow gradually increases to a value which is only slightly less than in the control state, in spite of the maintenance of the stimulus. This autoregulatory escape seen in the gastro-intestinal tract does not occur in all tissues. The mechanisms underlying autoregulatory escape in the gastro-intestinal tract have not been clearly defined but it may be the result of a redistribution of blood flow from the arterial vessels in the mucosa to the submucosa. This may be due to the differences in sensitivity of the different vessels to vasodilator metabolites which will build up during the initial period of reduced blood flow. On the capacitance side of the circulation, there is little autoregulatory escape so the constrictor effects are more maintained and mobilise blood from the gastro-intestinal tract into the general circulation.

An important characteristic of the hepatic circulation is that it receives two blood supplies; one from the hepatic artery which is at approximately aortic pressure (120/80 mmHg), and a second from the portal vein which is at a very much lower pressure (10–12 mmHg). The two streams of blood join and their pressures equalise as they enter the sinusoids. This equalising of pressures is probably brought about by the myogenic activity in the arterioles and precapillary sphincters near the sinusoids.

Blood flow in the portal vein increases if blood flow to the gastro-intestinal tract increases as, for example, occurs after a meal. Increases in liver metabolism will increase flow in the hepatic artery. There is also an interplay between the two inflows, such that, if flow via one system increases, flow through the other will decrease.

There is marked autoregulation in the arterial vessels of the liver and the effects of local metabolites seem to be the most important factor in controlling blood flow through these arterial vessels. There is much less smooth muscle in the portal venules so the major control of resistance is via the arterial vessels.

Increased discharge in the sympathetic nerves results in vasoconstriction of both the hepatic arterial vessels and the portal vessels but the hepatic arterial vessels show a marked 'autoregulatory escape' as it seen in the intestine. In the liver, this may have a protective function. As in the intestine, the effects of the nerves on capacitance may be more important than the resistance effects. Adrenaline, at physiological doses, normally causes a vasodilatation within the liver. Other hormones, especially gastro-intestinal hormones such as secretin and glucagon and bile salts and their metabolites, all influence liver blood flow but their precise mechanism of action remains unclear.

Further reading

Berne, R.M. & Rubio, R. (1979). Coronary circulation. In: *Handbook of Physiology, Section 2, The Cardiovascular System*, Volume 1, *The Heart*, pp. 873–952. American Physiological Society: Bethesda.

Donald, D.E. (1983). Splanchnic circulation. In: *Handbook of Physiology, Section 2, The Cardiovascular System*, Volume III, Part 1, pp. 219–40. American Physiological Society: Bethesda.

Heistad, D.D. & Kontos, H.M. (1983). Cerebral circulation. In: *Handbook of Physiology, Section 2, The Cardiovascular System*, Volume III, Part 1, pp. 137–82. American Physiology Society: Bethesda.

Knox, F.G. & Spielman, W.S. (1983). Renal circulation. In: *Handbook of Physiology, Section 2, The Cardiovascular System*, Volume III, Part 1, pp. 183–217. American Physiological Society: Bethesda.

Roddie, I.C. (1983). Circulation to skin and adipose tissue. In: *Handbook of Physiology, Section 2, The Cardiovascular System*, Volume III, Part I, pp. 285–317. American Physiological Society: Bethesda.

Shepherd, J.T. (1983). Circulation to skeletal muscle. In: *Handbook of Physiology, Section 2, The Cardiovascular System*, Volume III, Part 1, pp. 319–70. American Physiological Society: Bethesda.

West, J.B. (1979). Blood flow. In: *Respiratory Physiology — the essentials*. 2nd ed., pp. 32–50. Williams & Wilkins Co.: Baltimore.

7

REFLEX CONTROL OF THE CARDIOVASCULAR SYSTEM

The systems controlling the heart and circulation have two main functions. Firstly, they must achieve adequate perfusion of the different parts of the body. This is particularly important to organs such as the brain and heart whose blood supply must be maintained at all times. Thus, arterial blood pressure must be maintained. Secondly, the controlling mechanisms must be able to alter the output of the heart and the distribution of blood to different tissues to meet the differing needs of the body under a variety of circumstances. As was discussed in Chapter 5, this redistribution of blood is brought about by changes in the radius of the resistance vessels in the different circulations. This can be a result of local factors operating within the tissues, or changes in the activity of the nerves innervating the vessels, or the release of hormones, or a combination of all three.

All physiological control systems are made up of three basic components: the sensors, the central comparator and the effectors (see Figure 7.1). The variable to be controlled is measured by the sensor and information relating to this variable is then relayed to the central comparator. The central comparator then compares the actual level of the controlled variable with the level at which the variable should be maintained. It then causes the effectors to bring about changes in the variable to minimise the difference between the

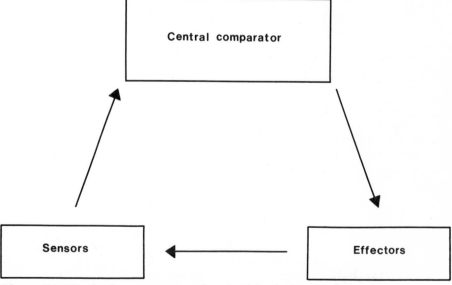

Figure 7.1. The basic components of a physiological control system.

recorded and predetermined level (or set point) of the variable. Modulation of the control system can take place at all of the three sites: the sensors (or receptors), the central nervous system (central comparator), and the efferent pathways (effectors). In this chapter, I shall describe some of the different reflex mechanisms which control the cardiovascular system. In the following chapters, I shall discuss the ways in which these different mechanisms can be modulated and integrated under different circumstances.

7.1 Arterial baroreceptors

Of the different groups of cardiovascular receptors, the arterial baroreceptors are the best documented. Baroreceptors are found in a number of sites in the body (see Figure 7.2), situated within the walls of large arteries. One important group of baroreceptors is found in the walls of the carotid sinus. The carotid sinus is a thinner-walled dilatation which lies at the bifurcation of the common carotid artery into the external and internal carotid arteries. This thinning of the wall results from a loss of some of the muscle from the tunica media. Other groups of baroreceptors are found elsewhere in the body, such as within the arch of the aorta and at the junctions of the subclavian and carotid arteries and of the thyroid and common carotid arteries.

The receptors are anatomically of different types, from diffuse nerve networks to more complex circumscribed endings. They are mainly situated in the deep layers of the adventitia of the vessel walls. It is not clear at present

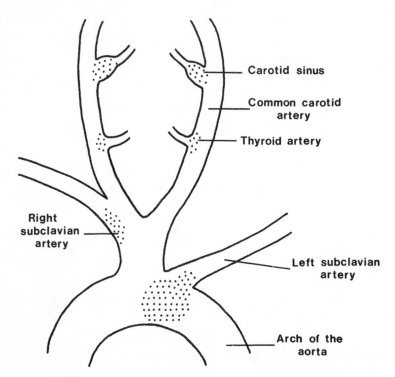

Figure 7.2. The main sites at which arterial baroreceptors are found in the body (indicated by shading).

how the receptors are arranged in relation to the muscle fibres. This is physiologically significant because if the receptors were arranged in series contraction of the smooth muscle would increase the stretch on the receptors whereas if they were arranged in parallel contraction would be expected to reduce the stretch on the receptors.

Baroreceptors respond to the amount of stretch on the artery walls. Thus, under normal circumstances, changes in the pressure perfusing the artery will result in changes in the activity of the baroreceptors. However, it has been shown that the direct stimulus to the baroreceptors is stretch of the vessel wall rather than pressure within the sinus. If the vessel wall is surrounded by a plaster cast, preventing it from distending, an increase in pressure within the vessel does not result in a change in the activity of the baroreceptors.

The properties of baroreceptors within the carotid sinus have been carefully studied in anaesthetised animals by perfusing the carotid sinuses with blood or an artificial physiological solution at different pressures and recording the discharge from the baroreceptor afferent fibres within the carotid sinus

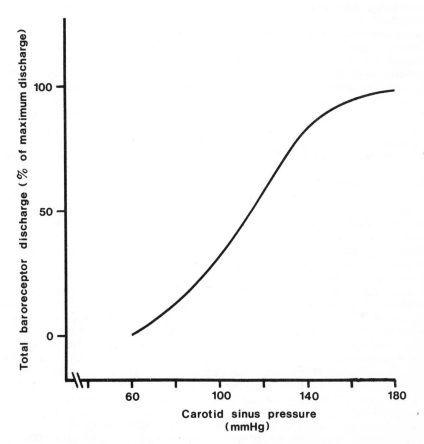

Figure 7.3. The relationship between the total discharge recorded from the carotid sinus baroreceptors, as a percentage of the maximum, and the pressure within the carotid sinus.

nerve. Using this technique impulses have been recorded from the baroreceptors at normal arterial blood pressure. Thus, the baroreceptors are said to be tonically active. Under normal circumstances increases in pressure within the carotid sinus result in increases in total baroreceptor discharge and, conversely, decreases in pressure result in decreases in total baroreceptor discharge. The relationship between the total discharge recorded from the carotid sinus baroreceptors and pressure within the carotid sinus can be represented by a sigmoid curve (see Figure 7.3). The relationship is linear over the range of pressures either side of the normal arterial blood pressure. Thus, at normal blood pressures, changes in pressure in either direction will alter the total discharge recorded from the baroreceptors. In contrast, at higher blood pressures, on the plateau part of the curve, changes in blood pressure result in very much smaller changes in baroreceptor discharge. Thus, the degree to which baroreceptor discharge can alter in response to a given change in blood pressure is highly dependent on the initial blood pressure.

As will be discussed further in Section 8.2, the set point about which this baroreceptor reflex operates is not fixed. It can be influenced by a number of factors including the time of day, the type of activity the subject is undertaking and the level of blood pressure over the preceding twenty minutes.

Baroreceptors within the carotid sinus respond not only to the static level of pressure within the sinus, but also to the rate at which the pressure is changing. If a steady pressure is applied to the sinus, the baroreceptors discharge in a regular manner. However, when a pulsatile pressure (a more physiological stimulus) is applied to the carotid sinus, the pattern of firing of the baroreceptors alters to a rhythm whose periodicity is determined by the frequency of the pulsatile signal applied to the sinus. The application of a pulsatile pressure results in a reduction in the threshold of some baroreceptors and hence a recruitment of baroreceptors, that is, an increase in the number of fibres which are active. Consequently, when pulsatile pressures are applied to the sinus, the total discharge recorded from the baroreceptors will increase. Thus, the discharge of the baroreceptors is influenced *in vivo* by changes in heart rate and pulse pressure as well as by changes in mean arterial blood pressure.

Recent studies in which recordings were made from individual baroreceptors have shown that the baroreceptors do not make up an homogeneous group. Two main groups of baroreceptors have been identified:
(1) small unmyelinated C fibres which are slowly-conducting,
(2) larger myelinated A fibres whose conduction velocity is faster.

The smaller unmyelinated baroreceptors mainly have an irregular pattern of discharge, even when subjected to pulsatile pressures, whereas the larger myelinated baroreceptors discharge with a pulsatile rhythm. Baroreceptors giving rise to the smaller C fibre afferents have a lower sensitivity, (that is, their discharge changes little in response to a change in pressure) and a higher threshold to stimulation, (that is, they start to discharge at a higher presure) compared to those giving rise to the larger A fibre afferents (see Figure 7.4). This means that, within the carotid sinus nerve, different fibres will be active depending on the pressure within the carotid sinus. At low blood pressures, more of the low threshold A fibres will be discharging but as carotid sinus pressure increases, more of the higher threshold C fibres will become active. Since the sensitivity of the A and C fibres also differs, the responses in the afferent nerves to a change in the carotid sinus pressure will vary depending on the proportion of A and C fibres which are active at any one time. At lower pressures, when the A fibres predominate, then the change

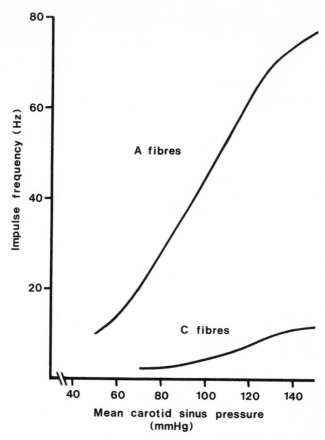

Figure 7.4. The relationship between discharge (impulse frequency) and mean carotid sinus pressure in the large, myelinated, baroreceptor afferents (A fibres) and in the small, unmyelinated baroreceptor afferents (C fibres) (From Yao & Thorèn, 1983).

in baroreceptor discharge in response to a given change in pressure will be greater than at high pressures when more of the less sensitive C fibres are active.

Differences have also been shown in the responses of baroreceptors at different sites, notably between the responses of the baroreceptors from the carotid sinus and those from the aortic arch. When recordings were made from groups of baroreceptor afferent fibres, those within the50Haortic arch had a higher threshold to stimulation and a lower sensitivity compared to those situated within the carotid sinus. However, when individual baroreceptor fibres situated in the two regions were subjected to the same stimuli and their properties were compared, no differences between the baroreceptors from the two regions could be detected. Aortic baroreceptors are also less sensitive to the rate of change of pressure than are the baroreceptors in the carotid sinus. The differences in the responses of groups of baroreceptors from the aortic arch and carotid sinus may simply be a reflection of the different pulse pressures to which the two groups of receptors are normally subjected. Pulse pressures in the carotid artery are far greater than those found in the thicker-walled elastic arteries such as the aorta (see Section 4.2.1). An alternative explanation might be that the proportion of baroreceptors giving rise to A and C fibres differs in the two regions. If, in the aortic arch, there was a higher proportion of C fibre afferents, this would explain the lower sensitivity and higher threshold to stimulation of aortic baroreceptors compared to carotid sinus baroreceptors.

Afferent fibres from the carotid sinus baroreceptors initially travel in the carotid sinus nerves and then in the glossopharyngeal nerves to the brain. Afferent fibres from the baroreceptors in the thorax are relayed to the brain within the vagal nerves. In some species, variable numbers of aortic arch baroreceptors may give rise to fibres which run in separate nerves, the right and left aortic nerves, which lie alongside the vagal nerves.

The primary afferent fibres from the baroreceptors synapse first within the nucleus tractus solitarius in the medulla. Connections are then made with the autonomic motor neurones of the sympathetic and vagal nerves through polysynaptic pathways. Studies in cats, dogs and primates have shown that the major output nucleus for the vagal efferent fibres is the nucleus ambiguus, which lies in the medulla. The preganglionic sympathetic neurones lie in the intermediolateral horn of the spinal cord.

The afferent fibres from the baroreceptors tonically exert an excitatory effect on the efferent neurones of the vagus and an inhibitory effect on the sympathetic efferent neurones. Thus, an increase in the baroreceptor discharge will produce an increase in the activity of the vagal nerves and a reduction in sympathetic efferent activity. Conversely, a decrease in the baroreceptor discharge will result in a reduction in the activity of the vagal nerves and an increase in sympathetic efferent activity.

Thus, qualitatively, the reflex effects of stimulating the baroreceptors can be predicted: a fall in the heart rate, a negative inotropic effect on the cardiac muscle (reducing its force of contraction), and a removal of the tonic vasoconstrictor tone exerted by the sympathetic nerves on the arterioles and veins, resulting in vasodilatation and venodilatation. There remains some controversy over the quantitative effects of baroreceptor stimulation on cardiac output. However, differing experimental observations can be explained in terms of differences in the resting levels of vagal and sympathetic nerve activity. There are also important differences in the responses of the different regional circulations to baroreceptor stimulation, the splanchnic and skeletal muscle vasculature being particularly sensitive.

In summary, changes in the arterial blood pressure are detected by baroreceptors which give rise to afferents which travel to the medulla and exert an excitatory effect on the vagal nerves and an inhibitory effect on the sympathetic nerves. Thus, the reflex effects of baroreceptor stimulation are bradycardia, a reduced force of contraction of the heart and dilatation of the arterioles and veins. These effects will lead to a decrease in the cardiac output and in the total peripheral resistance and, thus, a fall in the blood pressure. The role of this reflex in the regulation of arterial blood pressure will be discussed in Section 9.1.

7.2 Cardiac receptors

In addition to the arterial baroreceptors, there are also a number of different groups of receptors situated in the walls of the heart and in the tissues surrounding the heart. These cardiac receptors make up an even more varied group than do the baroreceptors. The different groups of receptors can be classified according to the type and size of afferent fibre they give rise to, where they are situated in the heart, and the modality of their adequate stimulus, for example, mechanical or chemical. When classified according to the type of afferent they give rise to there are three main types of cardiac receptor:

(1) receptors giving rise to large myelinated fibres which travel in the vagal nerves to the brain. One type of receptor of physiological importance is the so-called atrial receptor. The endings of these receptors are complex, but they are not surrounded by an accessory structure. They lie in the walls of the atrium and are concentrated at two main sites: on the left side of the heart at the junctions between the pulmonary veins and left atrium, and on the right side of the heart at the junctions between the right atrium and the venae cavae.
(2) receptors giving rise to small unmyelinated fibres (C fibres) which travel in the vagal nerves to the brain. These receptors are free nerve endings and are less complex than those giving rise to the larger fibres. They are very widely distributed throughout the thorax, for example, in the walls of the different chambers of the heart and in the pericardium.
(3) receptors giving rise to sympathetic afferent fibres of varying diameters which travel with the sympathetic efferent nerves to the spinal cord. These receptors also have a widespread distribution within the heart and large vessels and their fibres travel in the spinal cord to the brain within the spinothalamic tracts.

In view of the distribution of these different groups of receptors within the heart, there are considerable technical difficulties associated with adequately stimulating one group of receptors without producing changes in the discharge of other groups of receptors both within and outside the heart.

7.2.1 *Atrial receptors*
Distension, by means of small balloons, of the vein/atrial junctions has been used to stimulate the complex unencapsulated endings giving rise to the myelinated fibres. This technique also stimulates receptors which give rise to unmyelinated C fibres in the vagus and to sympathetic afferent fibres. However, since the reflex effects produced by distension are virtually abolished by cooling the vagal nerves (which removes the influence of the larger myelinated fibres) it can be concluded that the C fibres in the vagus and the sympathetic afferents contribute little to the reflex effects observed during distension. Using this technique, the reflex effects observed are an increase in the heart rate and urine flow but little significant effect on the inotropic state of the heart, respiration or peripheral resistance. The increase in heart rate is solely due to an increase in the activity of the sympathetic nerves to the heart, unlike the reflex changes in the heart rate induced by the baroreceptors which are due to a combination of changes in sympathetic and parasympathetic activity.

The mechanisms whereby stimulation of atrial receptors results in an increase in urine flow are still not completely established. There is evidence for a hormonal pathway. Plasma levels of anti-diuretic hormone (ADH), which increases reabsorption of water from the kidney, fall during distension, but it has also been suggested that a diuretic factor (as yet unidentified) may be involved. A neural pathway may also be involved since distension of the atrium has been shown to result in a reduction in the sympathetic efferent discharge to the kidney and an increase in the renal blood flow. Thus, changes in renal haemodynamics may also contribute to the increase in urine flow.

The reflex effects on the kidney accord with a role for these receptors in regulating extracellular fluid volume. The physiological role of the reflex changes in heart rate is less obvious, but may nevertheless be as important. As was discussed in Section 3.2.2, increases in heart rate result in a reduction in the time that the heart has to fill (the time of diastole) and, thus, in the end-diastolic volume. Thus, increases in heart rate may present the heart with a problem in that the filling of the heart may be compromised and, unless stroke volume can be maintained, there will be a reduction in cardiac output. However, such a mechanism may be useful in that if heart rate is increased in response to an increased venous return, since there is no associated positive inotropic effect, diastolic filling will be reduced so the size of the heart can be regulated. Therefore, it has been postulated that this reflex, in addition to regulating extracellular fluid volume, is also important in regulating the size of the heart. According to Starling's law of the heart (see Section 3.2.3), changes in the length of the muscle fibres over a limited range of muscle lengths regulate the force of contraction of the heart muscle. The reflex increase in heart rate produced by stimulation of atrial receptors, by reducing the filling of the heart, will reduce the length of the muscle fibres to within the range where their length can be regulated. A failure of the reflex response to stimulation of atrial receptors could result in over-distension of the heart.

7.2.2   C fibres

Stimulation of the free nerve endings which give rise to unmyelinated fibres within the vagal nerves results in a reflex bradycardia and hypotension, the so-called Bezold-Jarisch reflex. Both an increase in vagal activity and a reduction in the sympathetic efferent discharge are involved in this reflex response. In the past this reflex was evoked by the application of chemicals to the heart and was seen as being of more pathological than physiological importance. However, more recent work has suggested a more physiological role for these receptors. Some of these fibres are tonically active and alter their discharge in response to physiological stimuli. Increases in the pressure within the atrium (as will occur, for example, when venous return increases) or in the transmural pressure across the walls of the atrium (as will occur during the phases of respiration) both increase the discharge recorded from these receptors.

The threshold for stimulation of these receptors is higher than that of the myelinated atrial receptors but they still monitor changes in pressure which are within the physiological range. Receptors situated in the walls of the ventricles alter their discharge both in response to changes in left ventricular end-diastolic pressure and to changes in the inotropic state of the heart. These receptors often discharge during systole and yet their average rate of discharge is largely determined by the left ventricular end-diastolic pressure. Therefore they may be activated more when ventricular filling is increased, because the heart beats more strongly when the muscle fibres are stretched (Starling's law of the heart).

A major difficulty encountered in investigating these receptors is the unpredictable way in which they respond to a given stimulus. The same receptor may respond differently to the same stimulus at different times during an experiment. In contrast, receptors giving rise to myelinated fibres are very much more predictable in their response to a given stimulus.

Receptors giving rise to C fibres exert an inhibitory effect on the sympathetic nerves innervating the resistance and capacitance vessels, except the cutaneous veins. They have a particulary pronounced effect on the discharge of the sympathetic nerves to the renal vasculature and, thus, influence the excretion of sodium and water and the secretion of renin. Therefore, it has been suggested that these receptors, too, may play a part in the regulation of the extracellular fluid volume.

In addition to tonic effects on the sympathetic nerves, these receptors have been shown to be activated in a number of situations. For example, during a severe haemorrhage when the heart is contracting powerfully around an almost empty chamber, deformation of the myocardium occurs, and activation of the receptors. They are also activated during ischaemia of the heart resulting from occlusion of the coronary arteries. The reflex bradycardia and hypotension evoked under these circumstances have a useful role in that they reduce the work done by the heart and, hence, reduce the oxygen demand and blood supply required by the heart. There is also evidence of a reflex activation of the cholinergic nerves to the coronary vessels which would result in a dilatation of these vessels.

In addition to the free nerve endings described above, which can be stimulated by mechanical as well as chemical stimuli, there are a group of receptors in the heart which are stimulated by 5-hydroxy-tryptamine (5-HT). Stimulation of these receptors produces a pronounced hypertensive effect. One can speculate that this reflex may be important in removing blood clots which form in the coronary circulation. 5HT is released by platelets during haemostasis and the resultant reflex increase in the pressure perfusing the coronary arteries may be adequate to remove clots from the vessels in the heart.

7.2.3 *Sympathetic afferent fibres*

Sympathetic afferent fibres give rise to a variety of endings which are intermingled with the vagal endings throughout the heart. They are also found in the roots of the large vessels and in the tissues surrounding the heart. The fibres are of varying diameter and are both myelinated and unmyelinated. Some are silent and others are spontaneously active.

The discharge of the spontaneously active fibres is often related to mechanical events in the heart, either distension of the walls of the heart or contraction of the cardiac muscle. The discharge of these fibres can be altered by normal haemodynamic events, for example, changes in atrial pressure. They alter their discharge in response to both stretching of the cardiac walls and contraction of the cardiac muscle. The receptors of sympathetic afferent fibres, including those activated by mechanical stimuli, are also powerfully stimulated by a variety of chemicals, including bradykinin, veratridine, potassium and acids. They are also strongly excited during some pathological situations such as ventricular fibrillation and myocardial ischaemia.

The reflex effects of stimulating these receptors remain ill-defined. Recordings from sympathetic preganglionic neurones in the spinal cord have shown a variety of mainly excitatory responses to the stimulation of receptors giving rise to sympathetic afferent fibres. Local excitatory reflexes whose afferent and efferent pathways lie within the sympathetic nerves have been shown to exist in both the heart and in the carotid sinus region. Excitation of sympathetic afferents also inhibits the discharge of vagal efferent fibres, thus providing evidence for the existence of sympatho-vagal reflexes.

It is now generally accepted that the cardiac pain associated with angina or myocardial infarction is relayed to the brain in those fibres which travel within the spinothalamic tracts of the spinal cord. Within the spinothalamic tracts, there is considerable convergence between these sympathetic afferent fibres and somatic afferent fibres, and this may explain why a large number of patients with myocardial ischaemia have pain referred to the chest wall or the arms. There is also evidence that activation of these ascending systems involved in the perception of cardiac pain is prevented by an increase in the discharge of vagal afferent fibres. This may explain why, in some patients, myocardial ischaemia is not associated with cardiac pain, because the perception of pain will depend upon the relative degree of excitation of sympathetic afferent and vagal afferent fibres.

7.3 Other receptors

In addition to the arterial baroreceptors and the different groups of cardiac receptors, many other groups of receptors in the body can produce profound effects on the cardiovascular system.

Peripheral chemoreceptors can affect both the heart and blood vessels. In experimental animals, using conventional anaesthetics such as chloralose or barbiturates, and in which ventilation is controlled, the direct effects of stimulating chemoreceptors in the carotid body are bradycardia, a negative inotropic effect on the heart muscle and a vasoconstriction resulting from an increased discharge in sympathetic vasoconstrictor fibres. In the intact animal, these effects are over-ridden by the secondary effects resulting from the associated increase in ventilation (see Section 8.1). Stimulation of the chemoreceptors in the aortic body produces different effects on the heart, namely a reflex tachycardia and a positive inotropic effect on the cardiac muscle.

Stimulation of a variety of somatic and visceral afferents can result in a reflex increase in blood pressure. Thus, the number of different inputs to the brain which can potentially modify the cardiovascular system is immense. The following chapters deal with the ways in which these inputs are integrated and modified to produce a pattern of response which is appropriate for the situation in which the body finds itself.

Further reading

Coleridge, H.M. & Coleridge, J.C.G. (1980). Cardiovascular afferents involved in regulation of peripheral vessels. *Ann. Rev. Physiol.* **42**, 413–27.

Kircheim, H.R. (1976). Systemic arterial baroreceptor reflexes. *Physiol. Rev.* **56**, 100–76.

Linden, R.J. (1975). Reflexes from the heart. *Progress in Cardiovascular Diseases* **18**, 201–21.

Linden, R.J. (1979). Atrial reflexes and renal function. *Am. J. Cardiology*, **44**, 879–83.

Malliani, A. (1982). Cardiovascular sympathetic afferent fibers. *Rev. Physiol. Biochem. Pharmacol.* **94**, 11–73.

Scott, E.M. (1983). Reflex control of the cardiovascular system and its modification - some implications for pharmacologists. *J. Auton. Pharmac.* **3**, 113–26.

Thoren, P. (1979). Role of cardiac vagal C-fibers in cardiovascular control. *Rev. Physiol. Biochem. Pharmacol.* **86**, 1–94.

Yao, T. and Thoren, P. (1983). Characteristics of brachiocephalic and carotid sinus baroreceptors with non-medullated afferents in rabbit. *Acta Physiol. Scand.* **117**, 1–8.

8

CENTRAL CONTROL OF THE CARDIOVASCULAR SYSTEM AND MODULATION OF CARDIOVASCULAR REFLEXES

It must now be clear to the reader that the central nervous system receives a vast amount of information from different groups of receptors within the cardiovascular system. This information has to be integrated within the central nervous system and a response appropriate to the particular physiological circumstances elicited. The centrally-induced effects on the heart and circulation will be mediated largely by changes in the discharge of sympathetic and parasympathetic nerves and, to a much lesser extent, by the action of hormones. In this chapter, we are predominantly concerned with the mechanisms by which the outflow from sympathetic preganglionic neurones in the spinal cord and from vagal preganglionic neurones in the nucleus ambiguus of the medulla can be altered. Firstly, central drives on these neurones will be discussed, and then how the reflex responses to stimulation of different groups of receptors can be modified at a number of levels — at the receptor, within the central nervous system and along the output pathways — and how these different influences on the motor neurones are integrated to produce a pattern of response which is appropriate for the particular circumstance.

8.1 Control of the cardiovascular system by the central nervous system

Over the past twenty years there have been considerable changes in our views on how the cardiovascular system is controlled by the central nervous system. However, perhaps surprisingly, little of this information has found its way into text books of physiology until now.

The classical view argued for the existence of two reciprocating centres in the medulla, a pressor area concerned with increasing the activity of the sympathetic nerves and, thus, increasing blood pressure and a depressor area concerned with decreasing the activity of the sympathetic nerves and, thus, decreasing blood pressure. This theory was based on experiments carried out mainly in the 1930s and 1940s in which points within the brain stem were stimulated. Elaborate maps were then drawn to demonstrate the areas in which stimulation resulted in an increase or decrease in blood pressure. An example of a map obtained from one of the more recent, and often quoted, detailed studies is shown in Figure 8.1. The pressor centre was found to occupy an extensive region of the lateral reticular formation in the rostral two-thirds of the medulla, while the depressor centre included a greater part of the medial reticular formation in the caudal half of the medulla. At about the same time as these studies were being carried out, these same areas within the reticular formation were being cited as containing centres controlling respiration, as well as being responsible for somatic motor activity, for the

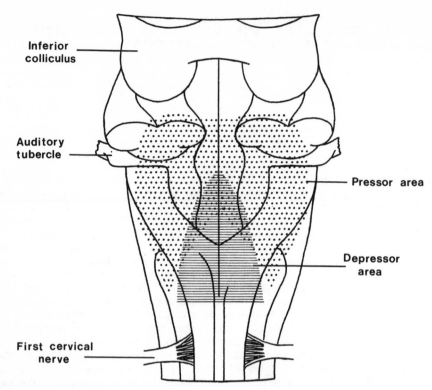

Figure 8.1. The positions of the pressor and depressor areas in the medulla of the cat (From Alexander, 1946).

states of sleep and wakefulness and for other autonomic functions, for example, motility in the gastro-intestinal tract.

The diversity of effects elicited by stimulation of these areas suggests that they are probably involved in a more general way in changing the level of activity of both the spinal motor neurones and the sympathetic nerves rather than being centres controlling blood pressure alone.

It is now clear that the medulla is not essential for the maintenance of the sympathetic discharge to blood vessels and, thus the maintenance of blood pressure. In both man and animals, following a recovery period after sectioning of the spinal cord, blood pressure is maintained and there is evidence that the sympathetic preganglionic neurones in the spinal cord are capable of discharging spontaneously even when all afferent inputs and influences from higher centres have been removed.

Normally, of course, discharge from the sympathetic nerves can be influenced both by afferent inputs entering the spinal cord at the same level and by tonic activity in descending pathways whose activity will also be altered by afferent inputs. Thus, the medulla does have an important role to play in the maintenance of sympathetic discharge to blood vessels but this role can be taken over by the spinal cord in the event of damage to the medulla. There is, at present, still a great deal of controversy over the location of, and the existence of pathways from, groups of neurones which influence the output from the sympathetic neurones. Groups of neurones whose rhythm of discharge closely resembles that found in the sympathetic nerves have been identified both in the medulla and the hypothalamus. There is also a suggestion that the area of the hypothalamus responsible for the integration of the alerting or defence reaction (see later in this section) may exert a tonic control over the sympathetic neurones via a pathway running through the ventral medulla. Certainly, neurones in the ventral part of the medulla can modify the activity of sympathetic neurones but whether these neurones have tonic activity or whether they are normally influenced from within the defence area remains a matter for debate. Numerous other pathways converge onto the sympathetic preganglionic neurones in the spinal cord but the neuroanatomical details of these pathways are outside the scope of this book.

Any cardiovascular control system, however, has to do very much more than just maintain the tonic discharge of the sympathetic nerves. Considering this, the classical view of medullary centres controlling blood pressure is naive. The control systems have to integrate a vast array of afferent information and influence the outflow from the brain to produce a pattern of cardiovascular responses which will vary depending on the circumstances. Thus, the modern view of cardiovascular control is far removed from the idea of medullary centres which control blood pressure and is instead concerned with the initiation of different patterns of cardiovascular response.

Investigations into the role of the central nervous system in the control of the cardiovascular system are technically difficult and the data obtained are often open to a variety of interpretations. However, it is now clear that areas exist within the central nervous system which are responsible for the integration of different patterns of response and that the hypothalamus has an important role to play.

One such pattern of responses which has been studied in some detail is the defence reaction. This alerting reaction, which is clearly seen in dogs and cats, can be evoked by a number of stimuli both from peripheral receptors and from within the central nervous system. The behavioural responses include piloerection, arching of the back, spitting and snarling. The associated cardiovascular changes include an increase in heart rate and cardiac output together with a redistribution of the cardiac output. There is a widespread vasoconstriction, reducing blood flow in low-priority circulations such as the splanchnic circulation, and an increase in the blood flow to skeletal muscles. This latter effect is, in cats and dogs at least, partly a result of the activation of sympathetic cholinergic vasodilator fibres which innervate the blood vessels in skeletal muscle. It has been suggested that this pattern of behavioural and cardiovascular responses is still present in man, even if the behavioural effects are disguised. However, there is little evidence to support a role for the sympathetic cholinergic nerves in primates.

Stimulation within a well-localised area of the brain (see Figure 8.2) running in a longitudinal strip from the hypothalamus through the mid-brain can produce both the behavioural and cardiovascular components of the defence or alerting reaction. The hypothalamus is essential for the initiation of the defence reaction, although there is some controversy as to whether these two components are initiated from the same area or two neighbouring areas. The amygdala, which is part of the limbic system, plays an important role in the integration of the cardiovascular changes associated with emotion, which include an alerting reaction. The amygdala provides an afferent input to the hypothalamus which is blocked by the use of traditional anaesthetics. Recent studies using anaesthetics which do not block this afferent input have

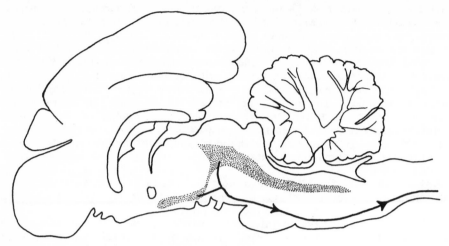

Figure 8.2. Diagramatic paramedian sagittal section through the brain of a cat. The shaded area represents the area involved in integrating the defence reaction in the hypothalamus and mid-brain (From Hilton, 1975).

shown that the defence reaction is elicited by stimulation of peripheral chemoreceptors. It may be that the defence area is not only responsible for the initiation of the full defence reaction as seen in cats and dogs but is also important in producing less extreme cardiovascular responses. For example, it has been suggested that the defence area is continuously active during the waking state, thus keeping blood pressure at a higher level than it is during sleep.

Studies on the control of the cardiovascular system in exercise suggest that there may be an area in the hypothalamus which generates the cardiovascular changes associated with exercise (see Section 9.3.1) in the same way as the defence area generates the alerting reaction. These cardiovascular changes are then modified by afferent inputs from the muscles and moving joints acting at the level of the spinal cord or at higher sites in the brain.

8.2 Modulation of cardiovascular reflexes

An observation of some of the patterns of response of the cardiovascular system to particular circumstances led to speculation that cardiovascular reflexes, particularly the baroreceptor reflex, could be modified. One of the first physiological situations in which it was thought that the baroreceptor reflex might be modified was exercise. During exercise, blood pressure and heart rate rise together, suggesting that the normal reflex bradycardia in response to the rise in blood pressure is suppressed. There is now evidence that at least one cardiovascular reflex, the baroreceptor reflex arc, can be modified by actions both at the receptors themselves and within the central nervous system.

A modulation of the stimulus/response characteristics of the baroreceptors can be produced in one of two ways (see Figure 8.3). Firstly, there could be a change in the threshold of the receptors, that is, the blood pressure at which the afferent fibres start to discharge. Changes in threshold will be seen as

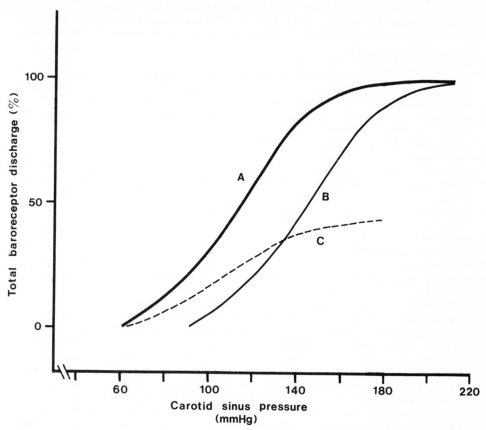

Figure 8.3. The effect a change in threshold and a change in sensitivity would have on the relationship between the total discharge recorded from the baroreceptors and the carotid sinus pressure. Curve A represents the control data, curve B shows a change in the threshold of the baroreceptor reflex and curve C shows a change in sensitivity of the baroreceptor reflex.

parallel shifts in the stimulus/response curves. Secondly, there could be a change in the sensitivity of the receptors, that is, the magnitude of the reflex response for a given change in the blood pressure. Changes in sensitivity will be seen as a change in the slope of the line relating response to stimulus.

8.2.1 *Effects at the receptor*

The carotid sinus region has a very dense innervation of sympathetic efferent nerves. Much work has been carried out to determine whether this efferent innervation of the sinus has a modulatory effect on the baroreceptors. Much of the early work on this subject produced controversial results but the possible role of these efferent fibres on the baroreceptor reflex arc is now becoming more clearly defined.

The sympathetic efferent nerves appear to have a number of effects on the baroreceptors. Firstly, stimulation of these noradrenergic nerves results, as would be expected, in a constriction of the carotid sinus. However, when the carotid sinus diameter is measured and comparisons of the baroreceptor afferent discharge are made at the same carotid sinus diameter both before and during sympathetic stimulation, stimulation of the sympathetic efferent nerves is shown to increase baroreceptor afferent discharge. Thus, the modulatory effects of the sympathetic nerves are not merely secondary to the reduction in the diameter of the arterial wall produced by sympathetic stimulation. Moreover, there is now some evidence that low frequencies of sympathetic stimulation may increase baroreceptor discharge by altering the electrophysiological properties of the receptors themselves.

The modulatory effects of the sympathetic efferent nerves on the baroreceptors do not appear to be uniform. The modulation is more pronounced in the unmyelinated rather than the myelinated afferent fibres. There is also evidence that, even within the myelinated fibre group, different afferent fibres respond differently to sympathetic efferent stimulation depending on their initial patterns of discharge.

Changes in sympathetic efferent discharge to the sinus can be evoked via the central nervous system but there is also evidence of local sympatho-sympathetic reflexes which can profoundly modify the level of sympathetic efferent discharge. These local reflexes, in which the afferent pathway is in the sympathetic afferent nerves (see Section 7.2.3) are usually excitatory.

In addition to the modulatory effects on the baroreceptors produced by the sympathetic efferent nerves, it has also been shown that the discharge of the baroreceptors is dependent on the blood pressure to which the receptors have recently been subjected. When blood pressure increases, baroreceptor discharge will initially increase but then, over a period of about twenty minutes, the discharge recorded from the baroreceptors will fall to a new lower level. When blood pressure falls, the discharge will initially decrease but then increase to a new higher value over a similar period of time.

This change in threshold, or resetting, of the baroreceptors in response to maintained changes in blood pressure has important implications for our understanding of the way in which the baroreceptors control blood pressure. It suggests that their major role lies in the detection of changes in blood pressure and that , in the face of a maintained level of blood pressure, they will adjust their own discharge accordingly. There is also evidence that the threshold of the baroreceptors will change as a result of structural changes in the vessel wall.

8.2.2 *Effects within the central nervous system*
Profound modulation of the baroreceptor reflex can occur not only at the level of the receptor but, also within the central nervous system. There are three main sites within the central nervous system at which a modulation of the baroreceptor reflex arc could take place. The first site is within the nucleus tractus solitarius which receives primary afferent fibres not only from the baroreceptors but also from a large number of other receptors including the arterial chemoreceptors and many of the cardiac receptors. The other two main sites at which modulation of the baroreceptor reflex arc could readily occur are the efferent preganglionic neurones which, for the vagal nerves, are within the medulla and, for the sympathetic nerves, are within the spinal cord.

The best-documented example of modulation of the baroreceptor reflex arc by a central mechanism occurs during the defence reaction. During electrical stimulation within a circumscribed area in the hypothalamus (from which the defence reaction can be evoked) the reflex effects induced by changing the pressure within the carotid sinus are completely suppressed. This suppression is mediated centrally rather than at some peripheral site since the reflex effects of stimulating the cut central end of the carotid sinus nerve are also suppressed during the defence reaction. Since, during the defence reaction, there is a suppression of all components of the baroreceptor reflex arc, it is thought that the modulation of this reflex during the defence reaction takes place soon after the baroreceptor afferent fibres enter the central nervous system. The most likely site for such a modulation is within the nucleus tractus solitarius, and there is some evidence for an interaction at this site. Stimulation within the hypothalamus has also been shown to inhibit the activity of the cardiac vagal motor neurones. This represents a possible pathway whereby the heart rate component of the baroreceptor reflex arc could be influenced without affecting the other efferent pathways of the reflex arc.

Stimulation within other areas of the brain, particularly within the hypothalamus and limbic system, can produce either an attenuation or a facilitation of the baroreceptor reflex arc. As might be expected, there remains disagreement between different groups of researchers as to the effects of stimulating at different points within the central nervous system. There are considerable difficulties in introducing a precise stimulus to one group of neurones in the brain without producing a spread of the stimulus and activating other nerve fibres which are running through the area.

Stimulation of these areas outside the defence area may affect only one component of the reflex. However, these modulatory effects on the different components of the reflex do not result merely from a summation of the direct effects of stimulation within the brain and the effects of baroreceptor stimulation. For example, stimulation within an area of the hypothalamus might produce, as a direct effect, a bradycardia but stimulation in this same area could also produce an attenuation of the bradycardia evoked by raising pressure within the carotid sinus. If the modulatory effects were merely a simple summation then one would expect, in this example, a greater not smaller bradycardia in response to baroreceptor stimulation during hypothalamic stimulation.

In addition to the modulation of the baroreceptor reflex arc produced during the defence reaction, there is also considerable evidence that the baroreceptor reflex arc is modified with the different phases of respiration. When recordings are made from cardiac vagal neurones in the nucleus ambiguus, an increase in blood pressure results in an increase in the discharge of cardiac vagal neurones, but only in the expiratory phase of respiration. During inspiration, an increase in blood pressure is ineffective in altering the firing of the vagal neurones which become hyperpolarised at this time. This modulation of the activity of the vagal cardiac motor neurones with respiration explains most of the changes in heart rate which occur during the phases of inspiration (sinus arrhythmia).

Another important site at which integration and modulation of the baroreceptor reflex arc can occur is at the sympathetic preganglionic neurones within the spinal cord. A number of pathways, both excitory and inhibitory, from higher levels in the brain can influence the activity of these sympathetic neurones. The baroreceptor-induced changes in sympathetic nerve activity are influenced by respiration in the same way as are the vagal motor neurones. However, this respiratory influence upon the sympathetic neurones is not as strong as in the case of the vagal neurones. There are also a number of possible interactions between these influences from higher centres and the segmental input to the sympathetic neurones from sympathetic afferent fibres, although as yet these interactions have not been defined.

8.2.3 *Interactions with other reflexes*

There is evidence that the discharge from a number of other receptors can modify the baroreceptor reflex. In animals anaesthetised with conventional anaesthetics an increased discharge from peripheral chemoreceptors will potentiate the baroreceptor reflex. However, when anaesthetics such as steroid anaesthetics (which do not block the afferent inputs from the amygdala to the hypothalamus) are used, stimulation of peripheral chemoreceptors evokes a pattern of responses which resembles the defence reaction (see Section 8.1). Stimulation of the defence area would be expected to attenuate the baroreceptor reflex. Cardiac receptors whose afferents travel in the vagal nerves also attenuate the baroreceptor reflex since, after vagotomy, there is a potentiation of the baroreceptor reflex. Thermal receptors and some groups of somatic afferent receptors can also modulate the baroreceptor reflex arc. Electrical stimulation which preferentially activates the small diameter somatic afferent fibres will attenuate the baroreceptor reflex. Thus, the magnitude of the reflex response to a given change in blood pressure can be markedly altered by the inputs from many groups of receptors.

The prevailing level of baroreceptor discharge can also affect the reflex responses produced by stimulation of other groups of receptors. As has been discussed earlier (see Section 7.2.2) receptors in the thorax giving rise to unmyelinated vagal fibres exert a tonic inhibitory effect on the sympathetic efferent nerves. This inhibition is far more marked when the pressure within the carotid sinus is low, that is, when the baroreceptor discharge is low, than when it is high. A high level of baroreceptor discharge also reduces the reflex responses evoked by stimulation of chemoreceptors and somatic afferent fibres. However, changes in the level of baroreceptor input do not appear to alter the cardiac responses to stimulation of atrial receptors.

There is also evidence for interactions both between baroreceptors from different sites and between baroreceptors giving rise to fibres of different diameters. When the baroreceptors in the cartoid sinus are stimulated together with baroreceptors in the aortic arch, the reflex response evoked is greater than the sum of the individual responses evoked by stimulation of the individual groups of baroreceptors. A similar facilitation has been shown between baroreceptors giving rise to myelinated and unmyelinated fibres. The simultaneous stimulation of myelinated and unmyelinated fibres from the same site produces a larger reflex response than would be predicted from the sum of the two.

8.2.4 *Modulation along the efferent pathway*

The final site at which reflex responses can be modulated is along the output pathways outside the central nervous system. Modulation and integration could take place both within the autonomic ganglia and at the autonomic effector junctions. There is now a lot of evidence that sympathetic ganglia play a much more complex role than simply to allow the passage of information through the ganglia. A great deal of integration can occur at this site. Similarly, modulation can occur at sympathetic neuroeffector junctions. The amount of transmitter released can be increased or decreased by the influence of a host of substances on the presynaptic endings. (see

Section 5.4). There is also scope for influencing the actions of the transmitter by effects on the post—synaptic membrane.

8.3 Summary

Thus, the modern ideas of cardiovascular control are very different from the classical view. Although arterial blood pressure must be maintained in order to achieve adequate perfusion, particularly of organs such as the heart and brain, the control systems have a very much more complex task to carry out than merely the maintenance of blood pressure. There is a mass of inputs to the brain which must be integrated to produce a complete pattern of cardiovascular responses appropriate for any particular circumstance. In the following chapter I shall discuss how these different mechanisms contribute both to the maintenance of arterial blood pressure and the provision of different patterns of response under different physiological and pathological conditions.

Further Reading

Abboud, F.M. (1979). Integration of reflex responses in the control of blood pressure and vascular resistance. *Am. J. Cardiol.* 44, 903—11.

Hilton, S.M. (1975). Ways of viewing the central nervous control of the circulation - old and new. *Brain Research* 87, 213—19.

Hilton, S.M. (1982). The defence-arousal system and its relevance for circulatory and respiratory control. *J. Exp. Biol.* 100, 159—74.

Hilton, S.M. & Spyer, K.M. (1980). Central nervous regulation of vascular resistance. *Ann.Rev. Physiol.* 42, 399—411.

Scott, E.M. (1983). Reflex control of the cardiovascular system and its modification - some implications for pharmacologists. *J. Auton. Pharmac.* 3, 113—26.

Spyer, K.M. (1982). Central nervous integration of cardiovascular control. *J. Exp. Biol.* 100, 109—28.

9

CARDIOVASCULAR CONTROL UNDER DIFFERENT CIRCUMSTANCES

In the preceding chapters, I described the different reflex mechanisms which influence the cardiovascular system, and explained how these reflexes can be modulated and integrated with the influences from higher centres. In this chapter, I shall speculate upon the relative importance of these different mechanisms both in the control of arterial blood pressure and in the cardiovascular responses to different physiological and pathological circumstances.

9.1 The control of arterial blood pressure

Arterial blood pressure will vary depending on the balance between the output of the heart and the condition of the blood vessels. This relationship can be expressed simply by the equation

$$\text{Blood pressure} = \text{Cardiac output} \times \text{Total peripheral resistance}$$

where the total peripheral resistance represents the total effect of the resistances to flow in all the blood vessels.

When considering the control of arterial blood pressure, it is important at the outset to differentiate between its short-term, that is, minute-by-minute control, and its long-term regulation. Different mechanisms are important in these two stages of control. Let us deal first with the short-term regulation of blood pressure, which can readily be illustrated by looking at the cardiovascular adjustments that occur in response to a change in posture or to a haemorrhage.

As discussed earlier (see Section 1.3), when a subject changes his position from the supine to the erect posture, the hydrostatic pressures within the vessels of the feet will rise and those in the head will fall. In the legs, veins which are not surrounded by dense fascial sheaths will distend. If the change in posture is not associated with active contractions of the muscles in the legs then blood will pool in the legs, thus reducing venous return to the heart. Consequently, cardiac output and blood pressure will fall. This pooling of blood in the veins will not occur to the same extent in the abdomen where interstitial pressures will also rise. In the vessels within the skull, the veins will not collapse because the pressure in the cerebrospinal fluid which surrounds the veins will also fall. However, as the external jugular veins leave the skull, they may collapse, since at this site pressure within the vessels will fall but the interstitial pressures remain unchanged. Within the carotid sinus, hydrostatic pressure will also be reduced so the stimulus to the baroreceptors will decrease. This, combined with the initial fall in blood pressure resulting from the venous pooling, will reduce the discharge from the baroreceptors.

The reflex-induced effects resulting from a reduced vagal efferent discharge and a removal of some of the inhibition of sympathetic efferent nerve activity will include an increase in heart rate of about 10 to 20 beats·min^{-1}, a positive inotropic effect on cardiac muscle and a widespread vasoconstriction. Total peripheral resistance will rise by about 30—40 per cent. This vasoconstriction is particularly marked in skeletal muscle and splanchnic beds but less pronounced in the skin. The increase in the rate and force of contraction of the heart and in the peripheral resistance compensates for the original fall in blood pressure. When the change in posture is passive, that is, the muscles in the legs are not contracting, there is considerable venous pooling. Under these circumstances, the increase in heart rate is not sufficient to compensate for the fall in stroke volume and cardiac output falls to a value of about 60—80 per cent of that in the supine position. Thus, since diastolic pressure increases but systolic pressure normally remains unchanged, pulse pressure will decrease. On standing, the reflex—induced increase in sympathetic efferent discharge also results in an increased output of renin from the kidney and an increase in the level of circulating catecholamines released from the adrenal medulla. These circulating catecholamines will tend to reinforce the actions of the sympathetic nerves.

The importance of the reflex increase in sympathetic activity can be demonstrated by blocking the actions of the sympathetic nerves. Tilting a subject from the supine position after pharmacological blockade of the sympathetic nerves will often result in his fainting since the reflex—induced sympathetic vasoconstriction no longer operates to maintain blood pressure and, hence, cerebral perfusion. Similarly, when standing motionless in the heat, the subject may faint. This is because the sympathetic vasoconstrictor activity resulting from reduced baroreceptor discharge is withdrawn due to the action of the hypothalamic regulatory centres in response to the raised environmental temperature.

The cardiovascular response to haemorrhage is another example where the baroreceptor reflex is an important mechanism in restoring blood pressure. In the short term, the reflex effects in response to haemorrhage are qualitatively very similar to those induced by a passive change in posture. As a result of the reduction in blood volume, cardiac output and blood pressure will initially fall. This will result in a reduced discharge from baroreceptors. Discharge from both myelinated and unmyelinated vagal fibres and from sympathetic afferent fibres originating in the atrium will also fall. During the haemorrhage, blood flow to the carotid and aortic bodies will be reduced and will result in an increase in the discharge from the chemoreceptors.

Occasionally, during a very rapid haemorrhage, the reflex-induced effects are a fall in the heart rate and blood pressure. These changes are mediated by the C fibres in the heart (see Section 7.2.2) and will not, of course, compensate for the drop in blood pressure resulting from the haemorrhage.

However, the usual reflex response to a haemorrhage is an increase in heart rate and in the force of contraction of the heart, a widespread vasoconstriction and venoconstriction, and an increase in ventilation. Thus, after a haemorrhage, patients breathe rapidly, have an increased pulse rate and their skin is white and may feel rather clammy. These changes are effected largely by an increased discharge in the sympathetic nerves, and by the release of circulating catecholamines. A withdrawal of vagal activity also contributes to the increase in heart rate. These reflex effects are mediated largely by changes in the discharge of the baroreceptors and chemoreceptors. The fall in the discharge from the atrial receptors will reduce heart rate but these effects are normally overridden by the arterial baroreceptors. However, the atrial receptors may contribute to the effects on the kidney. The contribution made by sympathetic afferent fibres remains unknown.

In the skeletal muscle bed, vasoconstriction is more predominent in pre-capillary than post-capillary vessels; thus capillary pressures fall and this will lead to an increased uptake of fluid from the interstitium into the blood (see Section 4.2.3).

In the kidney, the initial drop in blood pressure and the sympathetic vasoconstriction causes the release of renin which, via its actions on angiotensin, causes the release of aldosterone and, hence, an increased reabsorption of sodium from the kidney tubules. The reduced discharge of the baroreceptors and atrial receptors will result in the release of anti-diuretic hormone (ADH) and the retention of water. Thus, these mechanisms act to preserve sodium and water and, hence, increase the extracellular fluid volume. The release of renin, and its subsequent action on angiotensin, will also activate an area in the hypothalamus known as the 'thirst centre'. This will result in the subject feeling a strong sensation of thirst which will cause him to drink.

There are also metabolic effects in response to haemorrhage. Adrenaline release causes hyperglycaemia and the mobilisation of fatty acids. Adrenocorticotrophic hormone (ACTH) is released from the anterior pituitary and causes the release of cortisol which increases protein catabolism and gluconeogenesis. In the longer term, the loss of plasma proteins is compensated for by their increased manufacture in the liver. Red blood cell manufacture is also increased.

The importance of the sympathetic vasoconstrictor response was demonstrated unwittingly during the First World War. Because of the vast numbers of casualties, there were insufficient hospital beds available and some patients remained outside in the cold. Moreover, the only treatment available for those in hospital at that time was to be wrapped in blankets and given a hot drink. It was observed that those patients who were untreated stood a greater chance of survival. This observation can be explained by the interaction between the inputs from the baroreceptors and temperature receptors. In the patients left in the cold, the sympathetic vasoconstriction of blood vessels (particularly in skeletal muscle) induced via the baroreceptor reflex was reinforced by the increased sympathetic drive to blood vessels in the skin induced by the fall in environmental temperature. However, in the patients kept warm, the baroreceptor-induced sympathetic vasoconstriction would be opposed by the withdrawal of this sympathetic discharge to skin vessels because of the raised temperature, with the result that vasodilatation of the vessels would occur.

The initial compensatory mechanisms may not always be maintained. Pronounced vasoconstriction will lead to ischaemia of the tissues. In skeletal muscle particularly, this will lead to a vasodilatation induced by the accumulation of vasodilator metabolites (see Section 5.2). This vasodilatation affects the pre-capillary more than the post-capillary vessels and, therefore, will result in an increase in capillary pressure, an increased filtration of fluid and the subsequent accumulation of fluid in the interstitium. Consequently blood volume will fall. A loss of sympathetic tone to the venules and veins, and venous pooling may then follow. Blood pressure may not be maintained at a level adequate to ensure perfusion of the high priority organs (the heart and brain) and the patient will not survive.

Thus, the baroreceptors have a very important role to play in minimising deviations in blood pressure away from the set point. However, they do not appear to be important in the long-term regulation of blood pressure, that is, in determining the set point of the reflex. When blood pressure is measured continuously over the course of a day, the number of times the blood pressure

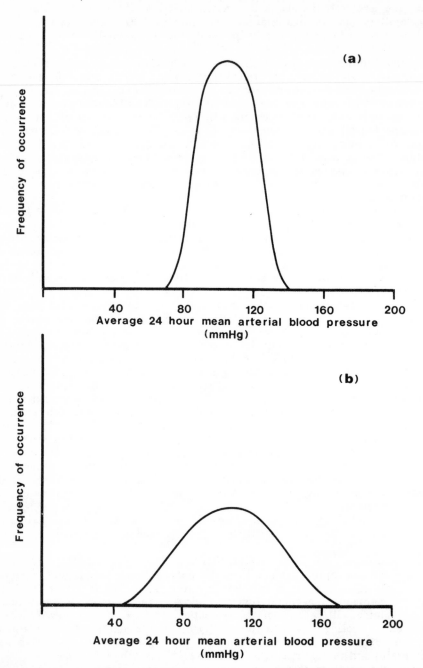

Figure 9.1. The frequency distribution of the blood pressure recorded during a normal 24 hour period
(a) in an intact dog and
(b) in a dog after section of the carotid sinus and thoracic baroreceptor afferent fibres.

is at a particular level can be displayed by means of a histogram. When the baroreceptors are intact, the range of blood pressures is quite narrow. This is evidence for the baroreceptors having an important role in returning the blood pressure to a set point when it is changed, for example, during changes in posture. However, when the baroreceptors are denervated, although the mean blood pressure remains the same, the range of blood pressures recorded is very much greater (see Figure 9.1). Thus, after baroreceptor denervation, the blood pressure is much more labile, but its mean value remains unchanged. In view of the recent observation that baroreceptors alter their threshold in response to a change in blood pressure which is maintained for as little as twenty minutes or so (see Section 8.2.1), it is difficult to see how these receptors could have a role in the long-term regulation of blood pressure. Thus, baroreceptors, although supremely important in short-term regulation of blood pressure, are of little importance in its longer-term regulation.

Normal values for systolic and diastolic pressure in man are usually quoted as 120 and 80 mmHg. However, the level of blood pressure is dependent on the age, race and sex of the individual, increasing with age, and generally being lower in women. It will also vary depending on the time of day and activity of the subject. Opinions differ among clinicians as to the upper limits of normal blood pressure for an individual and at what point treatment should begin to reduce blood pressure. There is considerable evidence that a sustained increase in blood pressure greatly increases the chance of suffering from cardiovascular disease and that this risk is reduced if blood pressure is lowered by treatment with drugs. Thus, some clinicians favour treatment with hypotensive drugs when the level of diastolic blood pressure at rest reaches values of 90–95 mmHg. Other clinicians, reluctant to prescribe drugs which will be taken over the course of years, argue that blood pressure is labile and is likely to be raised in people attending hospital as outpatients. Ideally, repeated measurements of blood pressure should be taken at rest on many different occasions and treatment started only when there is evidence that the rise in blood pressure is sustained.

9.2 Possible mechanisms causing the development of hypertension in man

The incidence of patients whose blood pressure is raised is very high in the western world. However, it is still far from clear what are the mechanisms which determine the set point about which the baroreceptors will operate to maintain blood pressure and how these mechanisms become deranged, allowing hypertension to develop. Theories abound and with each new study fashions seem to change. However, it is possible, from our knowledge of the mechanisms which can affect both cardiac output and peripheral resistance, to discuss the sorts of mechanism which may be important in the long-term regulation of blood pressure and to speculate on how changes in these mechanisms might lead to the development of hypertension. This approach should allow the reader to fit new theories into a rational framework and should avoid the problem of this account becoming out-of-date.

As discussed in Section 3.2.3, the two major determinants of cardiac output are the venous return to the heart, which will increase the end-diastolic volume, and factors such as the discharge of sympathetic nerves or the concentration of circulating adrenaline, which will reduce the end-systolic volume. Venous return will be increased either as a result of an increase in the extracellular fluid volume or as a result of decreases in the capacitance of vascular beds (such as the splanchnic bed) which result in a shift of blood towards the thorax. As discussed in Chapter 5, the major determinant of peripheral resistance is the radius of the pre-capillary resistance vessels. Thus, the long-term regulation of blood pressure involves mechanisms which regulate the extracellular fluid volume and which alter the radius of the capacitance and/or resistance vessels.

Extracellular fluid volume is mainly controlled by the kidneys and is achieved by regulating the outputs of sodium and water. In man, the intake of water can be regulated by the thirst centre in the hypothalamus and, in animals, mechanisms may exist which regulate the intake of salt. The renal mechanisms regulating the urinary outputs of sodium and water are complex and the details are outside the scope of this book. However, in principle, the outputs are determined by the balance between the amounts filtered and the amounts reabsorbed along the tubule. Filtration will be determined by the balance between hydrostatic and oncotic pressures at the glomerulus. Thus, mechanisms which either increase renal blood flow or alter the balance between the pressures in the afferent and efferent arterioles (see Section 6.6) will alter the filtered load. Changes in the amounts of sodium and water reabsorbed from the tubules can be affected by the redistribution of blood flow within the kidney and by the release of hormones. Aldosterone released from the adrenal cortex will increase the reabsorption of sodium from the tubule, and anti-diuretic hormone (ADH) will increase the reabsorption of water from the tubule. There may be other hormonal influences on tubular reasborption from the kidney, for example, a natriuretic hormone and a diuretic substance have been suggested, but these influences remain unclear.

Increases in extracellular fluid volume will be sensed by a variety of mechanisms (see Chapter 7). Stimulation of the receptors in the atrium which give rise to large myelinated vagal fibres results in an increase in urine volume which is, at least in part, mediated by a decrease in the concentration of ADH. Stimulation of cardiac receptors which give rise to C fibres will also alter the excretion of sodium and water. Stimulation of both these groups of cardiac receptors also decreases the discharge of sympathetic nerves innervating the kidney, which may alter both filtration and reabsorption. Osmoreceptors in the hypothalamus detect changes in the osmolality of the blood and these, too, influence the release of ADH. There are also sensors in the kidneys which indirectly detect changes in extracellular fluid volume and bring about the release of renin. A wide range of stimuli alters the release of renin including changes in blood pressure, in the discharge of the sympathetic nerves and in the flow of fluid along the distal tubule. Renin will ultimately cause the production of angiotensin II which not only may directly affect the blood vessels but will also cause the release of aldosterone. Often if extracellular fluid volume increases, so will blood pressure and the arterial baroreceptors will be stimulated also. Thus, a number of mechanisms exists to maintain the extracellular fluid volume within normal limits and these same mechanisms will, therefore, contribute to the long-term regulation of blood pressure.

The second major factor in determining blood pressure is the radius of the capacitance and, particulary, the resistance vessels. Structural alterations in these vessels or the deposition of material on the inside of the vessel wall may both reduce the internal radius of the vessels. Alterations in radius will also be brought about by changes in the level of sympathetic discharge to the vessel or changes in the level of circulating vasoconstrictor agents (see Sections 5.3 and 5.4). Some of the resting sympathetic tone originates at the preganglionic neurones in the spinal cord but there is also evidence for influences from higher levels in the central nervous system (see Section 8.1) and, of course, from a variety of peripheral afferents (see Chapter 7).

Although sectioning of the afferent fibres from the carotid sinus and aortic arch baroreceptors does not affect mean blood pressure, lesions in the nucleus tractus solitarius do result in a large increase in blood pressure. This could be because, even after sectioning the carotid sinus nerves and aortic nerves, a small number of baroreceptor afferent fibres remain intact whereas lesions in the nucleus tractus solitarius would destroy these remaining baroreceptor afferent fibres. However, there are many other explanations. The nucleus tractus solitarius receives inputs from a host of receptors, not only in the thorax but also in the neck and abdomen. The discharge from these receptors could influence blood pressure. In particular, the removal of the inhibitory effects on the sympathetic nerves which are exerted by the C fibres from cardiac receptors would increase blood pressure. It has also been suggested that the defence area in the hypothalamus (see Section 8.1), as well as initiating the 'flight or fight' response, may also excite the sympathetic neurones tonically and that this excitation varies depending upon the circumstances, for example, decreasing during sleep and increasing when the subject is alert.

Judging by the incidence of high blood pressure in the western world, the mechanisms which operate to maintain blood pressure often become deranged. In about 10 per cent of patients suffering from hypertension the cause is known, for example, it is associated with renal problems or toxaemia of pregnancy. The remaining large majority, in which the cause is unknown, is said to be suffering from essential hypertension, and a great deal of research has been done investigating the cause of it and finding suitable treatments. From the preceding discussion the possible causes should be clear. Either cardiac output or total peripheral resistance, or both, must be raised. Disturbances in the regulation of the extracellular fluid volume have been cited as explaining the development of essential hypertension. The association of hypertension and stress suggests that an increased sympathetic discharge may be a causative factor. One theory suggests that during stressful states intermittent bouts of sympathetic discharge, because they raise hydrostatic pressures in the resistance vessels, result in a hypertrophy of the smooth muscle of these vessels and, thus, a permanent narrowing of their walls. However, there is at present no clear consensus as to how hypertension develops. Genetic, dietary and environmental factors have all been implicated and it may well be that different defects in the controlling mechanisms are responsible for the development of essential hypertension in different individuals.

In the treatment of hypertension, prescribing habits vary as different drugs become fashionable. However, although the types of drugs used will vary over a period of time they must reduce either cardiac output or total peripheral resistance. Thus, diuretics, (which reduce extracellular fluid volume), drugs which reduce the level of sympathetic efferent discharge or which block the actions of the sympathetic nerves, drugs which inhibit the renin–angiotensin system and drugs which act directly on the smooth muscle of blood vessels to dilate them all have a rationale underlying their use as hypotensive agents.

9.3 Patterns of cardiovascular response and the integration and modulation of reflexes

In the cardiovascular responses to posture and haemorrhage the priority is the maintenance of blood flow to the brain and heart and this is achieved by a widespread activation of the sympathetic nervous system. However, the sympathetic nervous system is capable of much more discrete actions. One circumstance when the sympathetic nervous system acts in a discrete manner is when the atrial receptors giving rise to myelinated fibres are stimulated. Here, sympathetic discharge to the SA node is increased, to cardiac muscle and to blood vessels in skeletal muscle is unchanged and to the kidney is decreased (see Section 7.2.1). In the rest of this chapter, I shall describe the cardiovascular responses to a variety of circumstances in order to illustrate the different patterns of response of which the cardiovascular system is capable.

9.3.1 *Exercise*

One of the best-documented physiological circumstances is that of exercise. This is discussed in detail in another book in this series, so it will be considered only briefly here. During maximum isotonic exercise, such as running, oxygen consumption rises from a value of about 200–300 ml·min^{-1} when standing at rest to about 3–3.5 l·min^{-1}. This increase in oxygen supply is provided both by increasing cardiac output and by redistributing the blood to those parts of the body where it is most needed.

Cardiac output (see Section 3.2) is the product of heart rate and stroke volume. Heart rate will increase from a resting value of about 70 beats·min^{-1} to 180 beats·min^{-1}. Cardiac output will increase from 5 to 25 l·min^{-1}. Thus, the calculated stroke volume will increase from 70 to 140 ml per beat. About half of this increase in stroke volume is due to an increase in venous return, that is, an increase in the end-diastolic volume. In the erect posture, when a subject who is standing motionless starts to exercise, venous return will increase markedly because the pumping actions of the contracting muscles will reduce the venous pressures in the feet and, with the aid of the venous valves, blood will return to the heart (see Section 4.3). The remaining increase in stroke volume results from a reduction in the end-systolic volume, that is, the heart empties more completely. This inotropic effect is produced by the actions of the sympathetic nerves and by an increase in the level of circulating adrenaline. The associated increase in the velocity of contraction of the heart muscle will help to maintain filling of the ventricles by shortening the time of systole.

Associated with this increase in cardiac output are changes in the distribution of blood flow which will, of course, vary depending upon the type of exercise. Cerebral blood flow will be maintained, except, perhaps, if a subject exercises to exhaustion. The increased heart rate and force of contraction of the heart will increase the oxygen demand of the heart and consequently coronary blood flow will increase. Blood flow to the exercising muscles will increase in anticipation of exercise and at the start of exercise. This may result from the withdrawal of some of the sympathetic noradrenergic activity and, in animals, from the initiation of activity in the sympathetic cholinergic nerves. Both mechanisms will result in vasodilatation of the resistance vessels (see Section 5.3). Once the exercise is underway the build-up of local metabolites (see Section 5.2) will maintain the vasodilatation. Since these metabolites predominantly affect the pre-capillary resistance vessels, capillary pressure will rise and there will be an increased filtration of fluid from the capillaries and a subsequent accumulation of fluid in the interstitium. There will also be an increase in the number of capillaries perfused which, at rest, may represent only 10 per cent of the total. This increase in the number of capillaries perfused is important as it reduces the distance over which oxygen has to diffuse and increases the surface area across which diffusion occurs. Compensatory reductions in the blood flow to the renal and splanchnic circulations occur which are mediated via an increased sympathetic vasoconstrictor discharge. In addition, there are pronounced effects on the capacitance vessels thus mobilising blood. Initially, skin blood flow is reduced but, if body temperature rises as the exercise proceeds, then, in order to lose heat from the body, the sympathetic vasoconstrictor activity to the skin blood vessels is withdrawn and blood flow to the skin increases. Thus, in this type of exercise, systolic pressure will rise but diastolic pressure may fall.

In contrast, in isometric exercise, such as pushing against a fixed bar or holding a heavy weight, a different pattern of responses is seen. Here the muscles are contracting continuously, not phasically as occurs in isotonic exercise (such as running). This type of muscle contraction will occlude the blood vessels passing through the muscle. Thus, the resistance to blood flow in the skeletal muscles will rise and this, combined with the increased resistance in the splanchnic and other low-priority circulations, will produce a very large increase in both systolic and diastolic pressures.

This pattern of cardiovascular responses seen in exercise can be mimicked by stimulation within the hypothalamus and there appears to be a discrete area which is responsible for the initiation of this particular pattern of responses, in the way that stimulation of the hypothalamic defence region initiates the alerting reaction (see Section 8.1). A subthalamic area has also been suggested as the site controlling both the movements and cardiovascular changes during exercise. Any control from higher centres is greatly modified by afferent inputs from a variety of peripheral receptors, for example, from the moving joints and from receptors in the atrium responding to the increase in venous return. Local effects, as discussed earlier, are going to predominate in producing the hyperaemia found in the skeletal muscle and coronary circulations.

The cardiovascular response to exercise changes after training or a period of bed-rest. After a period of bed-rest of less than a month, maximal oxygen uptake decreases to about 2.5 $l·min^{-1}$, maximal cardiac output falls to 15 $l·min^{-1}$ and maximal stroke volume to 75 ml per beat. In contrast, training results in an increase in these values and in athletes of Olympic standard oxygen consumption may reach values of over 5 $l·min^{-1}$, cardiac output 30 $l·min^{-1}$ and stroke volume 165 ml per beat. Changes in maximum heart rate after bed-rest or training are small, if anything increasing after bed-rest and falling after training. Athletes have lower heart rates at rest and this is mainly due to an increased vagal activity to the SA node. The increases in stroke volume which occur during training are thought to result from an increase in the size of the heart rather than from any inotropic effect on the heart muscle. Capillary density in the cardiac muscle is also increased after training. If this large increase in the maximal cardiac output during exercise which is seen after training was not associated with a significant fall in total peripheral resistance, then blood pressure would increase sharply. In fact, blood pressure during exercise remains unchanged after training and, although total peripheral resistance during exercise does fall, the precise mechanisms whereby this happens are unclear. Presumably the effects occur at the arterioles within the skeletal muscle and they appear to affect only the trained muscles. It has been suggested that training results in a more complete withdrawal of the sympathetic efferent discharge to the blood vessels of the trained limb. This could be brought about by the inhibitory action of a local metabolite on adrenergic transmission. Capillary density within the skeletal muscle will also increase, but this will have little effect on the resistance to blood flow in the muscle.

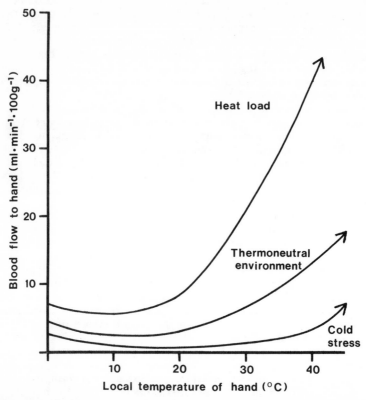

Figure 9.2. The effect on blood flow to a hand on its immersion in cold water during heat load, in a thermoneutral environment and during cold stress.

9.3.2 *Environmental temperature*

In response to a change in environmental temperature there is a characteristic pattern of cardiovascular responses. As temperature increases, sympathetic vasoconstrictor tone to the vessels of the skin is withdrawn in a sequential manner. Firstly, activity to the arterio-venous shunts in the ears and hands is withdrawn, followed by withdrawal of discharge to shunts in the feet. More general vasodilatation and venodilatation then follow. Thus, in this example, the sympathetic nerves are capable of acting in a highly discrete manner.

The magnitude of the response to a given change in local skin temperature will vary depending upon the heat stress of the body, as shown in Figure 9.2. These effects are not merely additive. If core temperature is high, then changes in local skin temperature will produce a very much more pronounced response to a rise in local temperature than will occur if core temperature is normal. Similarly, if core temperature is low an increase in local temperature will produce an attenuation of the local response compared to that which would occur when core temperature was within the normal range. This is an example of the way reflex responses can be modified depending upon the information the brain is receiving from other receptors.

9.3.3 *Ageing*

Modulation of cardiovascular reflexes occurs with ageing. There is evidence that the responses to stimulation of the baroreceptors induced by a variety of techniques including tilting or reducing lower body pressures (see Section 10.3) are altered in the aged. In the aged, the changes in heart rate and stroke volume on tilting are less than in the young. This attenuation of the reflex is associated with, and may be caused by, a reduced compliance, that is, a stiffening of the walls of the carotid sinus and aortic arch. Thus, for a given change in pressure, the arterial walls will distend less and, therefore, the stimulus to the baroreceptors will be less in the aged than in the young. The compliance of the veins will also be reduced in the aged, that is, the veins will be less distensible. This will mean that a manoeuvre such as tilting will not shift the central blood volume to the same extent as would occur in the young and, again, the stimulus to the baroreceptors would be reduced.

9.3.4 *Trauma*

The reflex response to stimulation of baroreceptors is affected by trauma. Haemorrhage produces a potentiation of the reflex whereas peripheral injuries such as fractures attenuate the reflex. The modulation occurring as a result of haemorrhage is similar to that produced by increasing plasma renin levels. Since plasma renin activity will increase after haemorrhage this is a possible mechanism for the potentiation of the reflex. In contrast, since the effects of peripheral injuries can be mimicked by limb ischaemia, there is evidence that the attenuation of the reflex after peripheral injuries is mediated by an increased discharge in afferent fibres from the damaged tissue.

9.3.5 *Eating*

Particular patterns of response are associated with eating. Stimulation of the 'hunger centre' in the hypothalamus initiates searching for food and increases food intake and gastro-intestinal motility and secretions. Associated with these changes are rises in blood pressure and heart rate and an increased vasoconstriction of the skeletal muscles together with an increased blood flow to the gastro-intestinal tract which may be a direct effect on the blood vessels or merely secondary to the increased activity in the gut.

9.3.6 *Sexual behaviour*

Activation of the parasympathetic nerves innervating the blood vessels in erectile tissue (see Section 5.3) can be initiated by stimulation of areas within the limbic system which are thought to be involved in the integration of the behavioural patterns associated with copulation.

9.3.7 *The diving response*

Another example of the interaction of different reflexes to produce responses of different magnitude occurs in the response to head immersion — the diving response. This response is particularly marked in diving animals such as the whale and seal during a prolonged dive, but it is also present in man, being particularly well-developed in trained divers, such as Korean women who dive for pearls. The classical diving response involves apnoea, a pronounced vagally-induced bradycardia, a fall in cardiac output and a widespread sympathetic vasoconstriction which affects even the skeletal muscle bed, in spite of the fact that the muscles are exercising and vasodilator metabolites are accumulating. There is also constriction of the capacitance vessels. Arterial pressure is maintained since the drop in cardiac output is balanced by the increase in total peripheral resistance, and the circulation is virtually converted into a heart—brain circuit. Coronary blood flow is reduced as the decrease in heart rate reduces the work of the heart and, hence, its oxygen need. The onset of the reflex is extremely fast, thus minimising the loss of oxygen to the peripheral tissues. This reflex enables diving mammals to remain immersed for very long periods. For example, whales can remain submerged for one or two hours even though their brains are as susceptible to hypoxia as are ours. Some diving animals, for example, ducks, whose dives are of a much more limited duration, do not normally show this response. During these very short dives, blood flow to skeletal muscle is increased and the pattern of responses resembles that of normal isotonic exercise (see section 9.3.1). However, during a prolonged dive, or if these animals are held under water, the classical diving response is seen.

The classical diving response is induced by stimulation of receptors in the mucosae at the back of the mouth, in the nose and in the pharynx, whose afferents travel in the trigeminal and glossopharyngeal nerves to the medulla. In man it can be produced by immersion of the face in cold water. The response is apparently organised within the medulla but there is evidence that higher centres are involved and that the response can be modified by influences from the cerebral cortex and hypothalamus. For example, the response can be conditioned and can be evoked in diving animals such as seals by threatening them. There is also evidence that, in man, the response to immersion can be modified. For example, it is attenuated during mental arithmetic, an activity which produces an alerting response similar to that evoked by stimulation of the hypothalamic defense area. There is also evidence that the response can be potentiated by an increased drive from the chemoreceptors which would occur, for example, during asphyxia. Stimulation of receptors in the walls of the airways by inflating the lungs removes these potentiating effects.

This diving response may be of considerable clinical importance. Face immersion, which evokes the diving response, has been successfully used to interrupt pathological tachycardia. It has also been suggested that the onset of the diving response, particularly if it is potentiated by an increased chemoreceptor discharge, for example, as occurs during asphyxia, may be the explanation for some types of sudden death. The increase in vagal activity to the SA node which is evoked during the diving response may be so intense as to stop the heart. This could explain the deaths of some asthmatics using a particular type of inhaler, deaths occurring during the introduction of a bronchoscope, some sudden deaths of swimmers attributed to drowning and the 'cot deaths' in neonates in which there is often evidence of mucus secretion in the upper respiratory tract. It may be that this reflex is particularly well-developed in some individuals and in some of the above cases, such as asthmatics, there is evidence of asphyxia. The knowledge that this reflex can be overridden by stimulation of lung stretch afferents can also be of clinical value since inflation of the lungs can be used to suppress some vagally-mediated bradycardias.

On removal of the stimulus to the diving response, there is a very pronounced 'off-response' in which blood pressure rises very steeply to values which may exceed 200 mmHg. This may be the cause of some cerebral vascular accidents in man.

If the diving response is found to be the mechanism responsible for some deaths it clearly illustrates the problems associated with trying to decide which physiological research will ultimately be of clinical relevance. Who would have thought that studies on the duck and seal during diving might aid us in our understanding of the most distressing sudden death syndrome in infants?

Further reading

Åstrand, P. & Rodahl, K. (1977). Regulation of circulation during exercise. In: *Textbook of Work Physiology* (Ed. P. Åstrand & K. Rodahl), pp. 170–205. McGraw Hill Book Company:

Blomqvist, C.G. (1983). Cardiovascular adaptations to physical training. *Ann. Rev. Physiol.* **45**, 169–89.

Daly, M.D. & Angell-James, J.E. (1979). The diving response, its possible clinical implications. *Int. Med.* 1, 12–19.

Gauer, O.N. & Thron, H.L. (1965). Postural change in the circulation. In: *Handbook of Physiology*, Section 2, The Cardiovascular system, Volume III, pp. 2409–40. American Physiological Society: Bethesda.

Little, R.A. & Stoner, H.B. (1983). The modification of homeostatic reflexes by trauma. In: *Shock Research* (Ed. D.H. Lewis & U. Haglund), pp. 101–7. Elsevier Science Publishers:

Rowell, L.B. (1983). Cardiovascular adjustments to thermal stress. In: *Handbook of Physiology*, Section 2, *The Cardiovascular System*, Volume III, Part 2, pp. 967–1023. American Physiological Society: Bethesda.

Sleight, P. (1983). Hypertension. In: *Oxford Textbook of Medicine* (ed. D.J. Weatherall *et al.*), pp. 13.258–13.278. Oxford University Press: Oxford.

10

ASSESSMENT OF THE FUNCTIONING OF THE HEART AND CIRCULATION IN MAN

In both clinical medicine and research, there are many techniques available to measure different physiological variables. The clinical techniques vary, not only from hospital to hospital depending upon the local expertise available, but also within any one hospital as new advances are made. A comprehensive account of all of these techniques is inappropriate for a short chapter in a text book for pre-clinical students. No attempt has been made to make this account comprehensive or to give sufficient detail to enable the reader to carry out the investigations himself. These skills will be acquired throughout a student's clinical training and practice.

This account is divided into three parts. In the first section, I shall consider the simple observations and measurements which would normally be carried out, often initially by a general practitioner or casualty officer, before referral to a cardiology unit. The second section will deal briefly with some of the more specialist investigations which may be carried out in a department of cardiology. The third section will discuss the tests which can be undertaken in man to investigate the autonomic control of the heart and circulation.

10.1 Initial examination

Careful questioning of the patient and an examination of the patient's medical history are the first steps towards a correct diagnosis. The patient may experience breathlessness at rest or during exertion. Dizzinesss on standing may reflect inadequate baroreceptor reflexes. The occurrence of pain, either at rest or during exercise may indicate an inadequate blood flow to a region; pain in the chest may result from an inadequate blood flow to the heart leading to cardiac ischaemia; intermittent pain in the legs, particularly during exercise (intermittent claudication), may be due to inadequate blood flow to the skeletal muscle in the legs.

Observation of the patient is also important. If the examination is carried out at a comfortable environmental temperature, then the colour and temperature of the skin may indicate the state of the peripheral vasculature. If the vessels are dilated then the skin will be redder and warmer than if the vessels are constricted when the skin will be pale and cold. There may be regional differences in skin colour or temperature which will reflect regional differences in the distribution of blood flow. An inadequate blood flow to one part of the body may result in cyanosis (a bluish colouration to the skin) only in that region. Changes in the condition of the skin, for example, loss of hair and brittle nails, may indicate a chronic arterial insufficiency. The presence of oedema will indicate an imbalance in the forces across the capillaries or changes in the permeability of the capillaries or venules.

10.1.1 *Arterial pulses*

An investigation of the arterial and venous pulses forms an important part of the examination. Following ejection of blood into the aorta, initially the inertia of the blood in the aorta prevents the immediate rise of pressure in the more distal parts of the arterial tree. However, this inertia is quickly overcome and the pressure pulse is then rapidly transmitted through the arteries by distending the vessel walls. The velocity of transmission of this pressure pulse along the artery wall far exceeds the velocity with which the blood travels along the arteries. The pulse wave can be felt at a number of places in the body. The main peripheral pulses which should be noted as part of the examination are the radial, brachial, carotid, femoral, popliteal, posterior tibial and dorsalis pedis pulses. The rate, rhythm and character of the pulse are normally assessed by palpation of the radial pulse at the wrist. However, the characteristics of a more central pulse, for example, the carotid pulse, will more closely resemble the aortic pulse. The pulse at the wrist is delayed and its volume is greater than that of pulses recorded nearer to the heart. A great deal of information about both the heart and circulation can be derived from a careful examination of the arterial pulses.

The pulse rate is counted over a period of at least half a minute. Measurements should not be made immediately upon palpating the pulse because any initial nervousness on the part of the patient will increase heart rate. In conditions such as atrial fibrillation, not all contractions will be strong enough for the pulse to be palpable at the peripheral arteries. In these situations, comparisons between the heart rate measured from the heart sounds and by palpation of a peripheral pulse should be made. The pulse rate will largely depend upon the balance between the activity in the sympathetic and parasympathetic nerves to the heart although it can also be influenced by circulating hormones (see Section 3.2.1).

The pulse can be described as regular or irregular. Some irregularities have a regular pattern, for example, the changes in heart rate associated with respiration (sinus arrhythmia). In other cases the irregularities have no fixed pattern and result from disturbances in the normal sequence of electrical activation of the heart (see Section 2.3.1.). Further information concerning abnormal rhythms can be derived from the ECG tracings (see Section 10.2.1).

The character or form of an individual pulse wave should also be examined. Changes in the form of the pulse can occur, for example, during stenosis or incompetence of the aortic valves.

The pulse pressure (the difference between systolic and diastolic pressure) gives an estimate of the volume of the pulse. This will depend upon the stroke volume and the compliance of the vessel walls. In older patients with normal stroke volumes, pulse pressure will be increased because of the reduced compliance of their vessel walls. Pulse pressures may also increase if cardiac output is raised.

The condition of the artery wall can also be assessed. In young healthy people the artery walls may not be felt as they are soft, but in older people the arteries are more easily palpable as they harden with age. In conditions such as arteriosclerosis, where the arteries become more rigid, the arteries feel hard and are tortuous.

An abnormal delay in the arrival of a pulse in one part of the body compared to another may indicate major abnormalities in the proximal vessels, for example, compression or constriction.

10.1.2 *Arterial blood pressure*

Normally the next measurement to make would be the systemic arterial blood pressure. This is routinely done using a sphygmomanometer which consists of an occluding cuff, a mercury manometer and a bulb with which the pressures applied to the cuff can be varied. The lability of blood presure with the time of day, posture, excitement and activity of the subject and the importance of repeated measurements to produce a reading of the blood pressure which represents a normal resting value have been discussed earlier (see Section 9.1).

Using a sphygmomanometer, an occluding cuff, to which varying pressures can be applied, is placed around the upper arm and the presence of blood flow distal to the cuff is established either by palpating the radial pulse (the palpation method) or by listening for the appearance of turbulent flow in the brachial artery (the auscultation method).

The palpation method is normally only used to estimate the systolic blood pressure. The pressure in the cuff is raised so that the radial pulse is no longer palpable and is then slowly lowered. The pressure in the cuff when the radial pulse can first be palpated is taken as the systolic pressure. Systolic pressure is normally under-estimated using this method compared to estimates made using the more sensitive auscultation method. Some cardiologists maintain that, with practice, diastolic pressure can be measured by palpation. This is done by continuing to lower the pressure in the cuff until a softening of the pulse is felt. However, this technique is rarely used.

The basis of the auscultation method is the recording of the noise produced when blood flow is turbulent. Again, the pressure within the cuff is raised so that it exceeds the systolic pressure and no radial pulse is palpable. Then a stethoscope is placed on the brachial artery and the pressure in the cuff is steadily reduced. When the pressure in the cuff exceeds systolic pressure the artery is occluded by the cuff and there is no blood flow to the arm. Hence, no sound is heard through the stethoscope. As the pressure is slowly lowered a sequence of sounds, the Korotkoff sounds, is heard. At the point when the pressure in the cuff is just less than the systolic pressure, blood will flow past the cuff in spurts with each heart beat. This blood flow is turbulent and therefore noisy. The pressure at which the sounds first appear is taken as the systolic pressure. As the pressure in the cuff is lowered, the sounds increase in intensity and finally become muffled. This latter point represents the transition of the blood flow from turbulent to laminar and, in Britain, this is normally taken to be the diastolic pressure. In some countries the point at which the sounds disappear is taken to represent the diastolic pressure.

In some hypertensive patients, the sounds disappear between systolic and diastolic pressure and then reappear. This is known as the 'silent gap' and its significance is unclear. If the cuff pressure is not initially raised above the systolic pressure, as assessed by palpation of the radial pulse, then the presence of the silent gap may lead to errors in the measurement of blood pressure.

Since the occluding pressure must be applied evenly around the arm, the use of a standard cuff in obese adults and in children could lead to inaccuracies in measurement so cuffs of different sizes are available.

A person experienced at this technique can measure blood pressure to within about 5 mmHg which is adequate for most purposes. The disadvantage of this technique is that it does not give an instantaneous read-out of changes in blood pressure. Consequently, it is unsuitable for use in circumstances where a beat-by-beat recording of blood pressure is required.

10.1.3 *Venous pulses*

The veins in the neck communicate directly with the right atrium. Therefore, estimating the mean pressure within the veins and the character of the pulse can give us valuable information about the mean pressure in the right atrium and the changes in right atrial pressure which occur with each cardiac cycle.

In a healthy subject, the mean hydrostatic pressure in the neck veins is approximately equivalent to the height of the clavicle above the heart so normally the neck veins are collapsed above the level of the clavicle. However, if atrial pressure is raised, the neck veins become distended and the pulsations are visible above the clavicle. In order to examine the venous pulse the patient's neck should be supported and reclined until the neck veins are visible. This will allow an estimate of the mean pressure in the veins to be determined.

Of the three waves on the atrial pressure pulse, (see Section 2.7) only the 'a' and 'v' waves may be seen on inspection of the jugular pulse. In young healthy subjects, these pulsations are not normally very prominent. However, the 'a' wave will become prominent when the resistance to filling of the right ventricle is increased or when the work of the right ventricle is increased, and will disappear if there are no active contractions of the atrium. If the tricuspid value is incompetent, then instead of the 'v' wave which represents filling of the atrium, there will be a large wave occuring during ventricular systole as blood surges back into the atrium.

Abnormalities in the sequence of electrical activity in the heart can be detected by comparing the jugular venous and carotid arterial pulsations. For example, if the normal passage of electrical activity across the heart is impeded, regular 'a' waves will be seen on the venous pulse but they will occur at a higher frequency than the carotid pulsations.

10.1.4 *Cardiac inspection, palpation and auscultation*

It is important that the chest wall be examined first for structural abnormalities which may cause a displacement of the heart or may be associated with the appearance of murmurs.

The lowest and most lateral point at which cardiac pulsations can be palpated is termed the apex beat (see Figure 2.10). The position of the apex beat may alter if the viscera surrounding the heart are diseased and consequently displace the heart or if the heart itself, particularly the left ventricle, becomes enlarged. If the left ventricle is enlarged, the apex beat is stronger and can be palpated over a larger area than normal.

The characteristics of the heart sounds, which are caused by closure of the heart valves, have been discussed earlier (see Section 2.7.1). Differences in the intensity of the sounds, abnormal splitting of the sounds or the presence of additional sounds or murmurs at various times during the cardiac cycle are very useful diagnostic aids.

10.1.5 *The peripheral vascular system*

Information about the state of the peripheral vessels can be derived from a number of simple tests. If the blood flow to a region is inadequate, capillary filling after lightly running a finger over the skin is often delayed. The condition of the arteries and veins in the eye can readily be seen using an ophthalmoscope.

The appearance of superficial veins not normally visible may result from the excessive pooling of blood in the veins. This could be caused by the failure of the venous valves, the presence of a thrombus in a deep vein or maybe associated with left ventricular failure. The efficiency of the venous valves can be assessed by a simple test known as the Trendelenburg test. The leg is elevated, venous return to the heart is increased and, thus, the veins empty. The long saphenous vein is then occluded proximally by applying pressure with the fingers. On standing, if the valves are intact and functioning normally, they should prevent the backflow of blood into the leg. However, if the valves are incompetent, the veins in the leg will fill with blood and become distended.

Using this array of non-invasive techniques, the experienced clinician is able to diagnose many cardiovascular disorders. However, more sophisticated investigations may be undertaken in the cardiology department, often as a prelude to surgery.

10.2 Examination in a department of cardiology

Within any one cardiology clinic a range of specialist investigations may be carried out on patients. The frequency with which particular investigations are used in a department will depend upon the interests and expertise of the members of that department. Some clinicians wish to have precise measurements of a range of cardiovascular parameters before making a diagnosis. Others will often diagnose and treat a patient without such precise data being available, using information derived from a number of qualitative investigations.

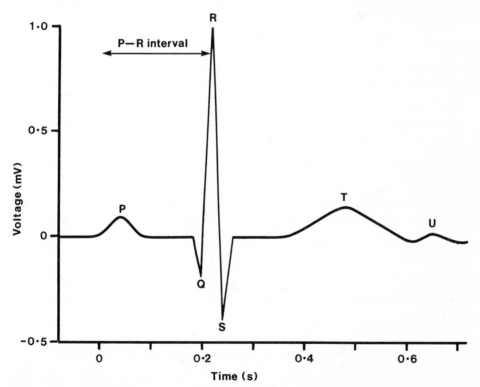

Figure 10.1. Diagrammatic representation of the waves of the ECG.

However, some investigations are common in all cardiology units. Routinely, most new patients will be given a full ECG investigation and a chest X-ray. An increasing number of these patients, perhaps as much as a third or half of them, will be examined using ultrasound techniques. In view of the frequency with which ECG and ultrasound investigations are carried out these will be considered first.

10.2.1 *The electrocardiogram (ECG)*

The initiation and spread of electrical activity in the heart is described in Section 2.2. The tissues of the body are good conductors of electrical activity so if electrodes are placed on the surface of the body, electrical activity generated in the heart can be recorded by means of a galvanometer.

The importance of electrocardiography as a technique for assessing electrical activity in the heart in man was clearly shown by Lewis in the 1920s using a galvanometer developed by Einthoven. Using electrodes attached to the limbs he obtained the classical recordings of the electrocardiogram (see Figure 10.1). The waves of the electrocardiogram represent the sum of the electrical activity in all the different cardiac muscle fibres. The P wave represents atrial depolarisation, the QRS complex (comprising the Q, R and S waves) represents ventricular depolarisation and the T wave represents ventricular repolarisation. Atrial repolarisation is lost within the QRS complex. In some recordings an additional wave, the U wave, is seen which is thought to represent repolarisation of the papillary muscles. The actual changes in voltage shown on the electrocardiogram are only a few millivolts compared to a change of about 100 mV when intracellular recordings are made directly from cardiac muscle cells (see Section 2.4). This is because the electrodes on the surface of the body are recording changes occuring a considerable distance away.

By convention, if the electrical impulse is travelling towards the electrode, the galvanometer will record a positive, or upward, deflection. Conversely, if the electrical activity is travelling away from the electrode, a negative, or downward, deflection will be observed. Since the mass of muscle in the left ventricle greatly exceeds that in the right, events occuring on the left side will dominate those occurring on the right side. Thus, the shape and direction of the different waves will vary depending upon the position of the recording electrodes. Consequently, twelve standard electrode positions or leads are used: three bipolar leads, in which electrodes are placed on two of the limbs, and nine unipolar leads in which only one recording electrode is employed.

With the three classical bipolar limb leads, two electrodes are used to measure the potential difference between two parts of the body: in lead I, electrodes are placed on the right and left arms, in lead II, on the right arm and left leg and in lead III, on the left arm and left leg. The deflection recorded using a bipolar limb lead represents the sum of the potentials recorded at the two electrode sites. These leads were used in classical studies and have yielded much information. However, they do have the disadvantage that changes in potential occurring at the different sites in the heart may be in opposite directions and so may not be detected when the sum of the changes is recorded.

When recordings are made from unipolar leads one electrode, the exploring electrode, is placed on the surface of the body at one of a number of points and the second, or indifferent, electrode is maintained at approximately zero potential by connecting electrodes from three limbs through a very large resistance. In the six chest leads, termed V_1 to V_6, the exploring electrode is moved progressively more laterally around the chest and the ECG is recorded

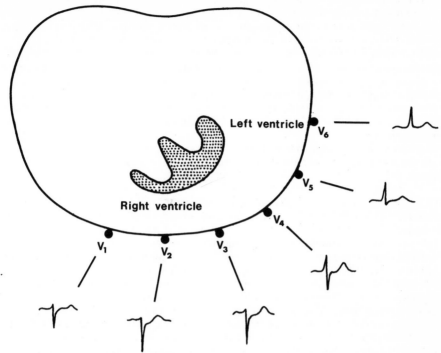

Figure 10.2. Cross-section through the chest to show the positions of the electrodes used in the six unipolar chest leads and the ECG traces obtained from each of these six leads.

from each of the six pre-defined chest positions (see Figure 10.2). In the three unipolar limb leads, the exploring electrode is placed on the right arm (RA), left arm (LA) and left leg (LF) respectively. Since the potentials recorded from the limb leads are often very small in magnitude, the augmented leads, aVR, aVL and aVF which produce larger potentials are normally used instead.

In physiology, the use of the ECG has allowed the normal sequence of electrical changes in the heart to be characterised in man. Clinically, the ECG can give valuable information about the sequence of electrical events occuring in the different parts of the heart, and structural abnormalities in the heart or damage to the heart muscle.

Changes in the sequence of electrical events in the heart can be detected by changes in the timing of the different waves of the ECG. For example, if there is an abnormal delay in the passage of electrical activity through the AV node (see Section 2.2.2), it will be detected as an increase in the P–R interval on the ECG.

Changes in the structure of the heart may be detected by changes in the size or shape of the different waves on the ECG. For example, several days after a myocardial infarction, the Q wave is more prominent and the T wave is often inverted. The leads with which these changes will be detected will depend upon the site of the infarction.

It is also possible to detect some gross structural abnormalities by estimating the electrical axis of the heart. This is the mean direction in which electrical activity passes across the heart and is obtained by summing the potential changes obtained using the three bipolar limb leads. Normally, the heart lies rotated towards the left in the chest. If the electrical axis of the heart is rotated towards the right, this might indicate a mechanical displacement of the heart; alternatively, it could mean that the electrical activity of the left ventricle was no longer dominant, because of either a loss of normal ventricular muscle or hypertrophy of the right ventricle. Conversely, an exaggerated rotation to the left could indicate hypertrophy of the left ventricular muscle.

Further details concerning electrocardiography are outside the scope of this book and the reader should consult one of the many clinical texts on the subject.

10.2.2 *Chest X-rays and ultrasound investigations*

Structural abnormalities of the heart and great vessels may be detected by examination of a chest X-ray, but the details will not be discussed here.

The use of ultrasound scanning (echocardiography) to detect a range of abnormalities is one of the most important developments in the measurement of cardiovascular parameters to have taken place over the past decade. This technique has the tremendous advantage of being non-invasive and is also less dangerous than X-rays. In all forms of ultrasonic examinations, a piezo-electrical crystal is intermittently excited and transmits bursts of high frequency sounds. These sound waves penetrate the tissue and are reflected back to a receiver. The time taken for the waves to return will depend upon the distance travelled, in the same way as the depth sounder on a ship works. Using this technique, the different layers of the heart muscle can be identified. Structures can be defined with an accuracy of about 0.1 mm. Thus, a very clear picture of the heart emerges, and the condition of the heart muscle and the valves can be examined. Calcified heart valves, for example, can be detected.

The movements of different parts of the wall of the heart and the valves during a cardiac cycle can also clearly be seen using echocardiography. If certain assumptions are made about the shape of the heart, then from ultrasound measurements an estimate of the end-diastolic and end-systolic volumes of the heart can be made. The use of 2- or 3-dimensional echocardiography increases the accuracy of such estimations considerably.

By injecting microscopic bubbles into the circulation, which strongly reflect ultrasound, the presence of shunts within the heart can be identified. In addition, ultrasonic techniques can be used to estimate the velocity of blood flow through the heart and great vessels. Two main types of flow meter are used. In one type, an ultrasound signal is transmitted diagonally across a vessel to a receiver. The sound is alternately transmitted in the same direction and in the opposite direction to the flow of blood. If the sound is travelling in the same direction as the flow of blood its velocity of transmission will be greater than if it is travelling in the opposite direction. The difference in the two velocities of sound transmission is a measure of the velocity of blood flow.

More commonly used flowmeters measure the shift in frequency between the transmitting and receiving signals (the Doppler shift). Again, an ultrasonic signal is transmitted across the vessel by a crystal. Some of this sound is reflected by the particles in the blood and is detected by the receiver. If the blood is not moving then the transmitted and reflected signals will have the same frequency. The velocity of blood flow is proportional to the difference between the frequencies of the transmitted and reflected sounds.

Doppler flowmeters are often used in combination with echocardiography so that the structure of the heart and vessels can be examined at the same time as estimates are made of the velocity of blood flow. Hopefully, continuing development of these techniques will ultimately allow cardiac output to be measured accurately by a non-invasive technique.

10.2.3 *Measurement of pressures within the heart*

Measurement of the pressures developed within the different chambers of the heart during the cardiac cycle is a widely-used and very useful specialist technique to assess the mechanical functioning of the heart. This is done by inserting catheters into the chambers of the heart which are attached to transducers which detect changes in pressure. The system used to measure the pressures must be capable of faithfully reproducing the shape of the pressure wave so must respond quickly (have a high frequency response). For the most faithful reproduction, the catheters themselves must be of a rigid material and must be as short, and of as wide an internal diameter, as possible. The frequency response of the system becomes even more critical when rates of change of pressure are being measured, for example, when the maximum rate of change of pressure in the left ventricle is being used as a measure of the inotropic state of the heart (see Section 3.2.3).

10.2.4 *Measurement of cardiac output*

Cardiac output can be measured in man by a number of techniques. At present, the most widely used are the direct Fick method and dilution techniques, although non-invasive techniques are being developed and their use is likely to increase.

10.2.4.1 *Direct Fick method*. This method ultilises the Fick principle for the measurement of cardiac output. The Fick principle states that the amount of a substance consumed or secreted by the whole body (or by an organ) is determined by the blood flow to the whole body (or organ) and the difference in the concentration of the substance in the arterial and venous blood. The principle can also be used to estimate blood flow to any region of the body (see section 10.2.6.1).

When the Fick principle is used for the measurement of cardiac output, it is assumed that cardiac output is equal to pulmonary blood flow.

$$\text{Pulmonary blood flow} = \frac{O_2 \text{ consumption ml} \cdot \text{min}^{-1}}{\text{Arterial } O_2 \text{ concentration ml} \cdot l^{-1} - \text{Venous } O_2 \text{ concentration ml} \cdot l^{-1}}$$

The oxygen taken up by the lungs is measured together with the oxygen concentration of the arterial and the venous blood. To estimate the arterial oxygen concentration a sample can be taken from any accessible artery but the sample of mixed venous blood is best obtained from the pulmonary artery. Thus, this technique has the disadvantage that it involves cardiac catheterisation.

10.2.4.2 *Dilution techniques*. A variety of dilution techniques is currently in use to measure cardiac output. A known amount of a substance, which stays

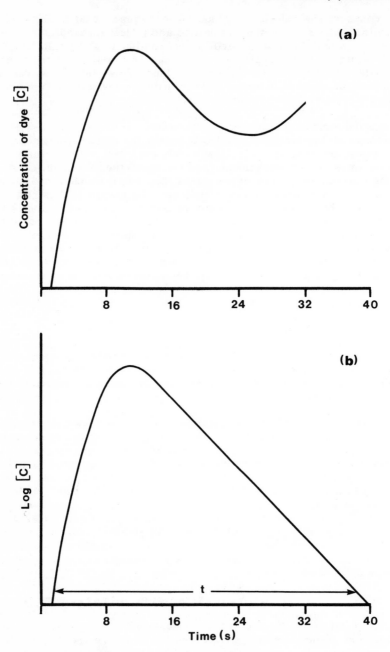

Figure 10.3. Estimation of cardiac output using the dye-dilution technique:
(a) changes in the concentration of the dye with time,
(b) the data from (a) replotted on semi-logarithmic paper to show how extrapolation of the declining exponential phase can be used to estimate the time for one passage (t).

in the blood stream, is injected and the average concentration of the substance over the period of a single circulation is measured at a sampling site. Cardiac output (CO) is calculated using the following equation:

$$CO = \frac{I \, g}{cg \cdot l^{-1} \times t \, s}$$

where I is the amount of substance injected, c is the average concentration of the substance and t is the duration of the first passage of the substance through the artery.

In the case of the dye-dilution method, the substance injected would be a non-toxic dye, normally indocyanine green. Blood is then withdrawn through a catheter implanted into an artery and the instantaneous concentration of the dye measured. As can be seen in Figure 10.3a, the concentration of dye increases, declines and then starts to increase again as the dye is recirculated around the body. To determine cardiac output, the average concentration of the dye during a single passage is required. Since there is an exponential decay in the concentration of the dye, when the curve is replotted on semi-logarithmic paper, the decay is linear and extrapolation of the line can be used to estimate the time for one passage (see Figure 10.3b). The area under this curve represents the product of the average concentration of the dye and the time for one passage.

Similarly, when radio-isotopes are used, the principle underlying the measurement of cardiac output is the same. A known amount of radio-isotope is injected and the average concentration determined by placing counters over the heart or lungs.

Thermal dilution is another variant of the dye-dilution technique and is increasingly used. An injection of cold saline is given and the temperature of the blood in the pulmonary artery measured by means of a thermistor attached to a catheter (Swan—Ganz catheter) inserted into the pulmonary artery. The shape and time-course of the changes in temperature of the blood in the pulmonary artery is similar to that of the dye concentration curve following dye ejection (see Figure 10.3) and cardiac output is calculated in a similar manner.

In practice, measurements of cardiac output are not often made unless cardiac catheters are already in place. In a patient who has already had catheters implanted, cardiac output is often measured using either thermal dilution or direct Fick techniques. In the latter case, a value for oxygen consumption is often assumed because many patients, unused to breathing into a mask, do not breathe normally so single measurements of their oxygen consumption are often unreliable.

10.2.5. *Other techniques for assessing heart structure and function*
The injection of radio-opaque contrast material into coronary vessels allows a picture of the coronary vasculature to be obtained (coronary angiogram). By injecting the contrast material into the chambers of the heart, similar techniques can be used to describe the internal dimensions of the heart and the heart valves.

The use of nuclear techniques is increasing. Nuclear angiography can be used to define the internal dimensions of the heart but is a less precise technique than contrast angiography for this purpose. Radioactive materials can also be used to demonstrate which areas of the myocardium are viable at any one time. Two different types of radioactive agents are used, those which are preferentially taken up by acutely injured cells ('hot-spot' scanning) and those which accumlate in viable, perfused myocardium but are not taken up by infarcted myocardium ('cold-spot' scanning).

Nuclear techniques can also be used to estimate the mechanical performance of the left ventricle. The injection of radioactive material into the heart allows an estimate of the left ventricular ejection fraction (the fraction of the end-diastolic volume ejected with each beat) to be made by a non-invasive method. Estimates of regional ventricular performance can be obtained by observing the movements of the ventricular wall.

10.2.6 *Measurement of blood flow*

A range of techniques is available for the measurement of blood flow to organs and tissues and particular techniques are used in particular organs and tissues. As in the earlier account of measurements in the heart, only the principles underlying some of the more widely used techniques will be considered.

The principles underlying the use of ultrasonic flowmeters have been described in section 10.2.2.

10.2.6.1 *Fick principle and clearance technique.* The use of the Fick principle in the measurement of cardiac output has been discussed in section 10.2.4.1. This principle can also be used to measure blood flow to an organ and in this case the content of the substance in the arterial and venous blood supply to that organ is measured.

This technique is used to measure the renal plasma flow and, in this example, the substance para-aminohippuric acid (PAH) is measured. This substance is not only freely filtered by the glomerulus but is also secreted into the tubules from the blood, so that the concentration remaining in the venous blood is very small. Thus, if it is assumed that the content of PAH in the renal vein is zero, the plasma flow can be calculated from the concentration of PAH in the renal artery and the amount of PAH excreted by the kidney. Thus,

$$\text{Renal blood flow} = \frac{UV}{P}$$

where U is the urinary concentration of PAH, $(mg \cdot l^{-1})$ V is the urinary flow rate $(ml \cdot min^{-1})$ and P is the plasma concentration of PAH $(mg \cdot l^{-1})$.

A similar technique can be applied to measure hepatic blood flow. The excretion of bromsulphthalein (BSP), which is removed almost solely by the liver, can be estimated. If the concentration of BSP in the hepatic artery and hepatic vein are measured, hepatic blood flow can be calculated using the Fick principle.

The Fick principle can also be used to estimate total cerebral blood flow in man. The subject breathes in a mixture of nitrous oxide (N_2O) in oxygen for ten minutes and during this time measurements of the concentration of N_2O in arterial and jugular venous blood are made and these values plotted graphically against the time at which the samples were taken. When the arterial and venous concentrations are equal, the amount of N_2O that has been taken up by the brain can be estimated. The integrated A-V difference for N_2O over the period of the test can be obtained from the graph. Thus, knowing the uptake of N_2O by the brain and the A-V difference, blood flow can be calculated.

10.2.6.2 *Dilution techniques.* A variety of dilution techniques are available in which the distribution of radioisotopes, radioactive microspheres, dyes or temperature gradients can be measured. These techniques can be used not only to measure the total blood flow to an organ but also to investigate the flow to different regions. For example, these techniques are used to investigate the intrarenal distribution of blood flow and the distribution of blood within the gut or the brain.

10.2.6.3 *Electromagnetic flowmeters.* This technique is the method of choice in many experimental studies and during some surgical procedures but it has the disadvantage of being an invasive technique. Two types of flowmeters are available, probes which are inserted into the vessel and collars which can be inserted around the vessel leaving it intact. The collar type is widely used, particularly in animal studies. Two small magnets are contained in the collar and are positioned on either side of the vessel. When blood moves through this magnetic field, it produces an electrical potential which is proportional to the velocity of blood flow. These flowmeters, when carefully calibrated, can produce a quantitative measure of blood flow through a vessel.

10.2.6.4 *Venous occlusion plethysmography.* This is one of a number of non-invasive techniques used to measure the blood flow to a limb. The extremity is enclosed in an airtight container, the skin junction is sealed, and the change in volume within the container is recorded. In order to measure the arterial inflow to the limb, venous drainage is temporarily occluded so the rate of increase of volume in the box gives a measure of the arterial inflow.

If a tourniquet is applied around the wrist or ankle, then much of the blood flow to the skin is prevented and an estimate of skeletal muscle blood flow to the forearm or calf can be obtained.

Instead of enclosing the extremity in a box, a mercury/silastic strain gauge can be used. This consists of a narrow flexible tube filled with mercury which is placed around the limb. As the limb volume increases, the strain gauge is stretched and the resultant change in resistance can be measured. These strain gauges are more convenient to use but are more difficult to calibrate and therefore less accurate than the more cumbersome box arrangement.

10.2.6.5 *Photoelectric transducers.* This simple non-invasive technique is used in man to measure blood flow in the finger or ear. A device is clipped over the finger, for example, and light is transmitted across the vessel to a photoelectric cell. The amount of light transmitted will depend on the volume of blood flowing through the finger.

10.3 Assessment of cardiovascular reflexes in autonomic failure

There is currently a great deal of interest in the assessment of autonomic failure in man. The following account will concentrate on the detection of disorders in the control by the autonomic nervous system of the cardiovascular system. However, since the autonomic system has such widespread effects within the body, associated changes in the function of other systems may also often occur. Patients may first visit their doctor with one or more of a range of symptoms, for example, impotence or dizziness.

Measurements of blood pressure, respiration, pulse rate and blood flow taken at rest may themselves indicate autonomic failure. For example, an

abnormally low blood pressure may indicate the loss of tonic sympathetic
vasoconstriction and venoconstriction, which occurs in chronic autonomic
failure. A number of different tests needs to be carried out in order to
determine the site of the disorder.

Failure of the sympathetic efferent nerves to respond to changes in
baroreceptor discharge can readily be detected by observing the change in
blood pressure when a subject stands. The initial investigation can be done
using a sphygmomanometer. If, on standing, systolic blood pressure falls by
more than 20 mmHg, further investigations are necessary. The changes in

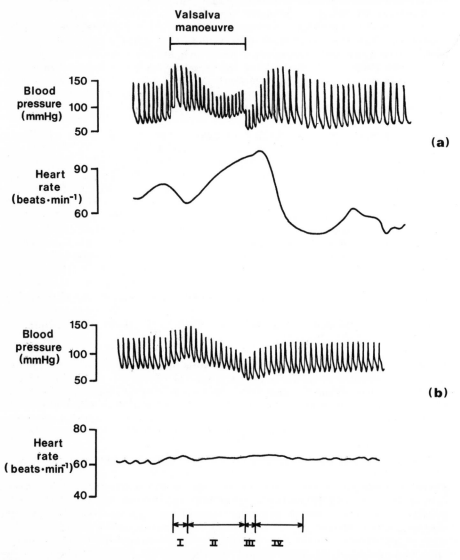

Figure 10.4. Cardiovascular response to a Valsalva manoeuvre in (a) a normal
subject and (b) a subject with autonomic failure. See text for explanation of
Phases I, II, III and IV.

blood pressure when a subject is passively tilted should then be measured. Blood pressure needs to be measured either by an arterial catheter attached to a manometer or by a photoelectric cell clipped over the finger (see section 10.2.6.5). The changes in heart rate with posture can easily be measured by recording the ECG. In patients with autonomic failure, the blood pressure will fall during the tilt, largely because of the lack of reflex contriction of the resistance and capacitance vessels. If only the sympathetic nerves are affected, some increase in heart rate, produced by a withdrawal of vagal activity to the heart, may still be seen on tilting.

The Valsalva manoeuvre is another simple, non-invasive test which can be used to detect autonomic dysfunction. In this test, the patient expires with a force sufficient to maintain a column of mercury at a height of 40 mm and then maintains this expiration for ten seconds. This will result in an increase in the subject's intrathoracic pressure. The response to a Valsalva manoeuvre in a normal subject can be divided into four phases (see Figure 10.4a). In phase I there is a transitory rise in arterial pressure and a fall in heart rate at the onset of the expiratory strain. This rise in pressure is normally attributed to the increased intrathoracic pressure compressing the aorta. In phase II there is a fall in blood pressure followed by a partial recovery of blood pressure and a rise in heart rate during the expiratory strain. The initial fall in blood pressure results from the decrease in venous return and consequent fall in cardiac output. The subsequent rise in blood pressure and heart rate is reflex-induced mainly by changes in the level of baroreceptor discharge. During phase III there is a further brief fall in blood pressure and a further increase in heart rate on ending the manoeuvre. This fall in blood pressure is thought to be due to the release of the compression on the aorta, that is, a reversal of the events occurring in phase I. Finally, in phase IV there is an overshoot of blood pressure accompanied by a fall in heart rate. Blood pressure rises here because venous return and cardiac output increase and the increased cardiac output is pumped out into vessels which are constricted. The fall in heart rate is again reflex-induced.

The changes in heart rate which occur during the Valsalva manoeuvre are mediated largely by changes in the activity of the parasympathetic nerves to the heart. The vasoconstriction is mediated by changes in the discharge of the sympathetic nerves to the blood vessels.

In some types of autonomic failure there is an abnormal response to a Valsalva manoeuvre. The partial recovery of blood pressure and the rise in heart rate during phase II are absent (see Figure 10.4b). This suggests an inadequate functioning of the cardiovascular reflexes (mainly mediated by baroreceptors). In addition, there is no overshoot of the blood pressure in phase IV (see Figure 10.4b). This latter observation can be explained in terms of the reduced level of vasoconstriction in the peripheral vessels into which the increased cardiac output is being pumped.

An abnormal response to tilting and to the Valsalva manoeuvre indicate a failure of the baroreceptor reflex somewhere along the reflex arc. Most commonly, these defects are found along the efferent pathway. Thus, other cardiovascular responses that are mediated by the autonomic nerves, for example, the response to exercise, stress or changes in temperature, may be abnormal. These effects are mediated largely by the sympathetic efferent nerves. Abnormalities in the functioning of the parasympathetic nerves to the heart can be assessed by recording the change in heart rate which occurs with each respiratory cycle during deep breathing. This sinus arrhythmia is mainly due to changes in the activity of the parasympathetic nerves to the heart although a small contribution is made by the sympathetic nerves (see section

8.2.2). The distribution of the nerves affected can be determined by looking at a range of responses, each mediated over different efferent pathways, and seeing which responses, and therefore, which nerves are affected. If the efferent pathways are intact, and yet the circulatory reflexes are affected, the defect will lie along the afferent limb of the reflex arc or within the central nervous system.

Other techniques to assess baroreceptor function are available. Although these techniques are not routinely used in clinical medicine, their use in research has yielded valuable information concerning baroreceptor reflexes in man. For example, the application of a negative pressure to the lower limbs is used to mimic the effects of standing. This produces a shift in the distribution of blood towards the lower part of the body and a subsequent compensatory reflex response. As with tilting and the Valsalva manoeuvre, this technique will alter the discharge from receptors in the heart as well as from the arterial baroreceptors.

In another test of baroreceptor function, which is now widely used in clinical research, the changes in heart period (the R—R interval on the ECG) in response to changes in blood pressure, induced by the injection of pressor drugs, are recorded. Arterial blood pressure is measured by an indwelling catheter. Each heart period is plotted against the systolic or mean pressure of the preceding pulse. Changes in the slope of this relationship are thought to

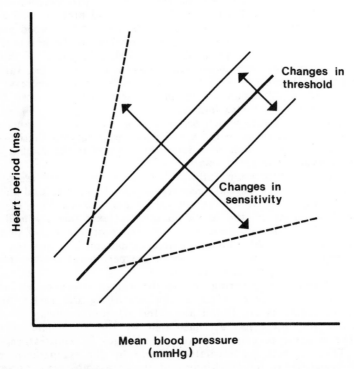

Figure 10.5. The effects of a change in threshold (——) and a change in sensitivity (---) on the relationship between heart period and blood pressure (——) (From Scott, 1983).

represent changes in the sensitivity of the reflex and parallel shifts in the line to represent changes in threshold (see Figure 10.5). The use of this technique for assessing baroreceptor function is based on the assumption that the relationship between heart period and blood pressure is linear. However, as has been discussed earlier (see Section 7.1), baroreceptors of different sizes and from different sites in the body have different thresholds and sensitivities so we are looking at not one but a whole array of stimulus—response curves. Thus, considerable care needs to be taken in interpreting the data obtained.

A more precise stimulus to a single group of receptors, that in the carotid sinus, can be applied by using the neck suction technique. In this non-invasive technique, the neck is surrounded by a box to which pressures can be applied. This allows the pressure within the carotid sinus to be varied and the reflex responses to changes in baroreceptor discharge studied in man.

Further reading

Bannister, R. (1983). Testing autonomic reflexes. In: *Autonomic failure* (ed. R. Bannister, pp. 52—63. Oxford University Press: Oxford.

Gibson, D.G. (1983). Echocardiography. In: *Oxford Textbook of Medicine* (ed. D.J. Weatherall *et al.*), pp. 13.34—13.41, Oxford University Press: Oxford.

Guyton, A.C., Jones, C.E. & Coleman, T.G. (1973). Methods for measuring cardiac output. In: *Cardiac Output and its Regulation*, pp. 21—134. W.B. Saunders Company: Philadelphia.

Miller, G.A.H. (1983). Cardiac catheterisation. In: *Oxford Textbook of Medicine* (ed. D.J. Weatherall *et al.*), pp.13.46—13.48, Oxford University Press: Oxford.

Rees, R.S.O. (1983). The chest X-ray in heart disease. In: *Oxford Textbook of Medicine* (ed. D.J. Weatherall *et al*), pp. 13.29—13.34, Oxford University Press: Oxford.

Rowlands, D.J. (1983). Nuclear techniques. In: *Oxford Textbook of Medicine* (ed. D.J. Weatherall *et al*), pp. 13.41—13.46, Oxford University Press: Oxford.

Rowlands, D.J. (1983). The Electrocardiogram. In: *Oxford Textbook of Medicine* (ed. D.J. Weatherall *et al*), pp. 13.48—13.58, Oxford University Press: Oxford.

Smyth, H.S., Sleight, P. & Pickering, G.W. (1969). Reflex regulation of arterial pressure during sleep in man: a quantitative method of assessing baroreflex sensitivity. *Circulation Res.* **24**, 109—21.

INDEX